My Imaginary Illness

A VOLUME IN THE COLLECTION
How Patients Think

WITHIN THE SERIES
The Culture and Politics of Health Care Work
edited by Suzanne Gordon and Sioban Nelson

A list of titles in this series is available at www.cornellpress.cornell.edu.

MY

A Journey into Uncertainty and

IMAGINARY

Prejudice in Medical Diagnosis

ILLNESS

CHLOË G. K. ATKINS

With a Clinical Commentary
  by **Brian David Hodges, MD**

Foreword by **Bonnie Blair O'Connor**

ILR Press *An imprint of*
Cornell University Press
Ithaca and London

First published 2010 by Cornell University Press

Printed in the United States of America

Library of Congress Cataloging-in-Publication Data

Atkins, Chloë G. K. (Chloë Gwyneth Katharine), 1965–

  My imaginary illness : a journey into uncertainty and prejudice in medical diagnosis / Chloë G. K. Atkins; with a clinical commentary by Brian David Hodges; foreword by Bonnie Blair O'Connor.

     p. cm. — (The culture and politics of health care work. How patients think)

  Includes bibliographical references and index.

  ISBN 978-0-8014-4887-4 (cloth : alk. paper)

  1. Myasthenia gravis—Diagnosis.   2. Somatization disorder—Diagnosis.

3. Diagnosis—Social aspects.   I. Hodges, Brian David, 1964–   II. Title.

III. Series: Culture and politics of health care work. How patients think.

  RC935.M8A85   2010

  616.7'442—dc22   2010013374

Cloth printing   10 9 8 7 6 5 4 3 2 1

I would not have survived this journey without the love and support of two extraordinary women: A.N.F. and A.L.M. They believed me when most thought me to be worthless, unstable, and incurable. My life and this book would not have been possible without them. My four children have also played an incalculable role in my survival and have endowed my life with a joy that I had never imagined possible—they too deserve credit for this tome's existence.

I came to explore the wreck.

The words are purposes.

The words are maps.

I came to see the damage that was done

and the treasures that prevail.

—ADRIENNE RICH, "Diving into the Wreck"

Contents

Editor's Note

This book is the second volume in our collection, How Patients Think. The inspiration for this collection was Jerome Groopman's book *How Doctors Think*, an interesting exploration of the way doctors have been socialized to think about patient care and the mistakes they can make because of that socialization. As Brian David Hodges points out in his clinical commentary at the end of this volume, Groopman—albeit with empathy and good will—seems to ask patients to adapt to, not merely understand, this medical thinking process.

In 2008, we, as editors of the Culture and Politics of Health Care Work series, launched How Patients Think to give patients a voice and to create a much needed dialogue among doctors, nurses, other clinicians, and patients. Our goal is to use each book as a forum in which patients and clinicians can bridge some of the gaps that often separate them. Each book in the collection presents the narrative of a patient. In this narrative we learn how patients think about disease and illness and their encounters with the health care system. We invite a health care expert—in this case the medical educator and ethnographer Bonnie Blair O'Connor—to begin framing the narrative in a foreword. The book is then concluded by a clinical commentary by a physician, nurse, or other clinician who reflects on some of the meanings and lessons of how patients think about a particular illness or set of encounters with the health care system.

Chloë G. K. Atkins's book is a perfect example of what we have to learn from listening to how patients think about their experiences. Her book focuses on the process of diagnosis and its power over both patients and doctors. She raises critical issues about what it means to be sick, to have that sickness named, and to be cared for in a complex technological medical system. In essence, this book is about a patient's struggle for what I have come to think of as a "good enough" diagnosis, one that allows the patient to be treated seriously rather than stigmatized, to be cared for, and to find some relief from her suffering.

SUZANNE GORDON

June 2010

Foreword

BONNIE BLAIR O'CONNOR

Much press has been devoted to how physicians, nurses, and other clinicians acquire and apply their knowledge and skills, how they interact with one another as coordinated professionals, and how they relate to and communicate with patients and their concerned family members in the setting of (especially, serious) illness and the care and treatment it requires.

This book is the second in a collection from the Cornell University Press series on the Culture and Politics of Health Care Work that focuses on "How Patients Think": how they experience their illnesses and the changes these make in their lives; how they seek, experience, and evaluate the assessments and treatments they receive; what helps, hinders, cures, or heals (for there is an important difference between the latter two); how they go on in the face of setbacks and disappointments; how they come to accept and make peace with what cannot be changed.

The books in this collection offer insight and constructive feedback for health-care professionals and educators, patients, family members, and friends of the chronically disabled or ill. They humanize the lives of patients and caregivers alike, and help us all come to understand one another other better as people in predicaments.

My Imaginary Illness recounts a lengthy struggle that includes many failures of efforts to diagnose and treat a strange and increasingly debilitating disease by clinicians both kind and empathic and distant to the point of hostility. Yet it is not a vehicle for "doctor-bashing" or bitterness. Reading the book as a career medical educator, I understand the physicians and nurses who are burdened by the expectation of society and their own professions that they should be able to "fix" anything and by their deep frustration with the baffling nature and apparent intractability of their patients' problems. Reading the book as a social scientist and medical ethnographer who takes what patients say seriously, I see an account of a severely disabling, yet medically contested, condition that appears to defy diagnosis, to the profound frustration of the patient. It is a tale of perseverance and problem solving that reveals along the way some worrisome fault lines in our health-care culture, and the strains in current professional training models and work conditions that underlie them.

Virtually everyone knows someone who has a health-care horror story: problems and delays in diagnosis or treatment; oversights and complications that should never have happened; wrong-site imaging or—worse—surgery; harried and unresponsive nurses; distant or abrupt physicians; clinicians who seem to be missing in action when the time comes to explain test or consultation results and their implications for treatment. So common are these and other errors of commission and omission that they are prime targets of hospitals' quality improvement initiatives, of regulatory mandates, and of a strong and growing international patient-safety movement.

Many of us have also felt frightened, ignored, belittled, accused, dismissed, or deeply and painfully humiliated by health-care professionals on whose knowledge, skills, and mercy we have depended when we were sick. These stories often remain private. They are not the focus of QI and patient-safety investigations, and they are so terribly personal and discomfiting that this variant of the story may be told only to a scant few intimates—if we can bear to articulate it at all.

Few of us know anyone who has even come close to what Chloë Atkins has suffered and survived through the development and idiosyncratic course of a chronic degenerative disease that eluded proper diagnosis, as well as anything resembling effective treatment for twenty agonizing years. That so many of the health-care professionals Atkins encountered were stymied for so long by her symptoms is frightening, but also explainable: the symptoms were uncommon, and there were no recognizable patterns on which to hang a definitive diagnosis. That so many were so cruel beggars comprehension.

When we enter the health-care system with serious symptoms, we come in with a dread of the devastating diagnosis, tempered by hope that our problem is trivial, or at least treatable. Perhaps an equal dread that many of us feel is of the experience Atkins recounts: that our problems will not be medically decipherable and will therefore be pronounced to be "all in our heads." This may be more true for women than for men, as a substantial body of research shows that women are disproportionately subject to this judgment. The poorly disguised disapproval that typically accompanies the delivery of this opinion reveals our society's continued conceptual separation of mind and body in illness, and our ongoing cultural stigmatization of the "mental" side of the divide.

Since the professional fields of medicine and nursing, and our health-care system as a whole, are products of that same society and overarching culture, the psychological label is also an early warning sign of trouble ahead for the patient. Once it is pronounced and written in the record, the patient has a second full-time job: the struggle to find and connect with clinicians who will not see her, from before they meet, through the lens of her preexisting "rap sheet." The psychological label creates a serious two-way impediment to trusting patient-clinician relationships. Yet trusting relationships are essential to unbiased assessment, to wide-ranging exploratory thought processes that strive to accommodate all of the objective *and* the experiential data, and ultimately to achieving a workable diagnosis in confounding, complex cases.

In this poignant personal-experience narrative, Chloë Atkins has portrayed the suffering of the patient who is subject to unsuccessful and even injurious treatment at the hands of a sizeable cast of physicians and nurses over a long period of time. The great majority of these people truly meant well; but they nevertheless both directly and indirectly caused physical, mental, and emotional harm and hugely increased the suffering Atkins experienced. The contrasting portraits of the genuinely engaged and caring clinicians she encountered are notable for the rush of relief and gratitude she felt for their empathic ministrations and their matter-of-fact acceptance of the patient's lived experience.

What can we learn from these behaviors, as health professionals and educators, as ordinary citizens? The astute clinical commentary provided by Dr. Brian Hodges illuminates much of what lies behind the kind of psychologizing and rejection that Atkins repeatedly met during her twenty-year quest for diagnosis and treatment. Hodges explains empathically—and without casting aspersions on either the reality of the author's medical crisis or the frustrations of her erstwhile care givers—why clinicians flee from patients with complex, chronic, and degenerative diseases; and reveals the professional, personal, and emotional quandaries in which such clinicians may find themselves. He does not excuse these behaviors, but he helps us understand them, and demonstrates how health professionals' educations and work cultures could be modified to ameliorate them.

Our current systems of medical and nursing education are in many ways antithetical to the raising of merciful healers, and Hodges offers realistic suggestions for enhancing clinical education and training to address the deeply human needs of clinicians and patients alike. Diseases do not come into the hospital in Little Red Wagons: they come in human beings, with all of their marvelous and challenging complexity, their infinite variability of presentations and responses to treatments, and their always unique selves. Hodges proposes a realistically attainable health-professional education and culture that would enable clinicians to engage both the diseases they treat and the people who experience them: to provide for healing, as well as medical treatment.

As Hodges also notes, Chloë Atkins's story can in places be a very rough read. There is anger in it, and despair—both appropriate to her situation; there are grim details, abandonment, and terrible treatment by some clinicians. Yet there are also perseverance and acceptance, kind-hearted clinicians, and steady, supportive love. And after all that, there is even a happy ending, though the serious disease is not cured. What the author was seeking for those twenty long years was not, after all, a cure: it was a diagnosis. Not an end to her symptoms, but a place to begin their proper treatment.

My Imaginary Illness should be read by physicians, nurses, and health-care professionals of every stripe, preferably early in their training and at intervals thereafter. It should be read by patients who have soldiered on through difficult diseases and still more difficult treatment; by people who have felt frightened and abandoned by those whom they have trusted to care; and by neighbors, friends, and family members of those who struggle with chronic and complex ills. No institution that internally purports, or publicly advertises, to provide "patient-centered care" should feel confident in making that claim unless its administrators and staff have first read and responded to this and similar narratives of patients' real experiences, both triumphant and troubling.

Acknowledgments

This book is a memoir that recounts certain scenes and omits others. This has been done to maintain narrative coherence and flow rather than to obscure or mislead. In this sense, it is not an encyclopedic recounting of every occasion but rather a pastiche of events in order to provide an understanding of what transpired.

Moreover, I've made every effort to safeguard the identity of all those involved. My aim is not to pillory or laud any single individual but to chronicle moments and conversations so that readers may be provoked to think, discuss and, (perhaps) criticize the way we view and confront illness, culturally, and, the way we treat it, medically.

This book has had a long gestation. It has taken many years (more years than I might have wished) to bring it to publication. As such, there are innumerable people who have had a hand in its current incarnation. Even as I thank those who have helped me down this arduous path, I am sure that I inevitably overlook individuals who have helped me complete this journey. I offer my apologies and my gratitude to them in advance.

I was fortunate that my political science doctoral supervisory committee at the University of Toronto encouraged me to explore narrative forms of scholarship. Consequently, portions of this book find their origin in my dissertation on political theory. Professors Ed Andrew, Joseph Carens,

Philip Hebert, and Jennifer Nedelsky provided unflinching and stalwart support even as my health flagged and it seemed I might not survive my PhD, let alone complete it.

During a Fulbright postdoctoral fellowship at Cornell University Law School, I encountered three remarkable colleagues: Martha Fineman, Risa Lieberwitz, and Ruth O'Brien. They have generously mentored me. Their guidance has indelibly sculpted my thoughts and writings ever since.

I am grateful to the Killam Trust's Resident Fellowship at the University of Calgary, which gave me a semester's break from teaching to do the final editing of this book. Cecelia Cancellero, my literary agent, was an early backer of this project. I am also greatly indebted to Suzanne Gordon, the series editor for Cornell University Press, whose professionalism, knowledge, and advice improved the original manuscript immeasurably. She also reconceived this project into its current form—that is, by including a physician commentator to provide a clinical perspective on my autoethnographic critique of my medical experience.

Normally, an author restricts her acknowledgments to those who have been involved in the writing of the book, however I would like to thank those clinicians who have had a direct role in my survival and thus the book's completion: doctors Christopher Atkins, Brian Goldman, Eric Kotzer, Colleen McGillivray, Jerry Tennenbaum, Sylvia Hidvegi, Brian Kavanagh, Ged Lippert, Peter Leung, Vincy Yam, and Keith Brownell, as well as several occupational and physical therapists and nurses who believed in and treated my symptoms. They have either literally saved my life or have worked to maintain my quality of life. Without them, this book, and I, would simply not be here.

Over the years, one individual, Alison Fisher, who has known me since my early childhood, has stood by me regardless of my circumstances. Finally, my spouse, Aruna Mitra, has read every word of this book a multiplicity of times. Her editorial skill and unflagging enthusiasm for my work provided both psychological and very concrete support for this prolonged project. As well, my four children, Justin, Alisha, Zephyr, and Callum, have all variously supported and endured its very long creation—at times, they have had to set aside their own needs by putting up with my crotchety moods, my distractedness, and my insistence on having a temporal and physical "room of my own" in which to think and write.

In sum, I owe many people in completing this book. I only hope that my efforts here match in some way the confidence and encouragement that they placed in me. Any errors, oversights, and deficiencies that may appear in the text, however, are mine alone.

Introduction

Sometimes it occurs only once, but sometimes twice or more often in a day. I might be sitting at my desk typing an e-mail, walking the length of a corridor on my way to lecture, or skiing with my family in the brisk air of a snowy day in the mountains, but the feeling is always the same. It envelops me and then it gently subsides. Initially, the impulse is so strong that I can momentarily sense my chest walls collapsing and oxygen-starved tissues burning as my body craves fortitude and air. And then the sensation passes.

At least once a day, sometimes more often, the inevitability of my own demise strikes me. Quite simply, there isn't a day that I don't think about dying. This has been happening for over a decade, and I presume it will continue until the day I really do die.

At first I found this stealthy and chronic reminder of my mortality enervating and demoralizing. It plagued me. An aimless jitteriness seized me, and I existed in a formless twilight of indecision and nihilism. And then, after several months, the oppression lifted. I began to find solace in the flitting of these dire sensations and images. The omnipresent awareness of my death freed me to live more fluidly. Although I am not religious, I came to embody the phrase from the Psalm of David: "Yea, though I walk through the valley of the shadow of death, I will fear no evil." I know each day to be a blessing.

You might think that my ongoing epiphany is hypochondriacal and Pollyanna-ish—and, on the surface, it is—but it arises from a crucible of experience that has marked me indelibly.

For more than a decade, from the age of twenty onward, I became progressively more ill and paralyzed. Despite the chronicity and increasing seriousness of my symptoms, physicians could find nothing wrong with me. Their inability to find a physical cause for my debilitating symptoms led to the pronouncement that my symptoms must be psychosomatic. Doctors insisted that I was unconsciously (and some even believed, consciously) making myself ill. Because I was estranged from my parents, my family situation served to confirm my physicians' diagnosis. I became the embodiment of an ancient Greek paradigm of hysteria morphed into late twentieth-century psychobabble. In medicine, psychogenic diseases are now variously called Briquet's syndrome, conversion reaction, somatoform disorder, or somatization disorder. But the underlying presumption is much the same: the patient (usually female) expresses unresolved psychic trauma or conflicts (which are often sexual) in bodily symptoms, for which no organic cause can be found. Ironically, according to the paradigm, the more the patient is adamant that her symptoms are real, the more clinicians presume that they are purely the result of intrapsychic phenomena. Moreover, doctors believe that such patients achieve some sort of secondary gain in acting out a sick role—they garner sympathy from friends and family, collect disability pensions, and become the focus of others' attention.

While many may think this is a relatively rare diagnosis, medical journals report that up to 50 percent of doctors' visits are the result of "psychological" or "stress"-induced problems. In other words, according to medical experts, psychogenic illness and pain are extremely common. The vast majority of us are presumed to experience it at some point in our lives.

What makes my experience unusual is the severity and frequent recurrence of my symptoms as well as the fact that my illness took place not only in Canada, a country with a national health system, but also in the United States, a country with a primarily private system. My many bouts of extreme weakness and complete paralysis, which at times required me to have resuscitation and life support, were nonetheless chalked up to psychological imbalance. Ironically, as I became more and more seriously ill, I received less and less medical support. It became impossible for my family doctor to find a consulting neurologist or internist to follow me medically. And I only sporadically obtained respiratory, physical, speech, or occupational therapy to help with my increasing disability. I was prescribed muscle relaxants, antidepressants, and narcotics (many of which had adverse effects) and was sent home. This, even after I became quadriplegic and eventually too weak to even chew and swallow food. My voice flagged and I choked on liquids, which caused pneumonia. I was often fed by a nasogastric tube, but even this method of liquid nourishment resulted in problems because my stomach's absorption capabilities at times all but ceased. On several occasions I was admitted to an intensive care unit (ICU) because my paralysis and weakness had become so profound that my diaphragm and chest muscles could not expand or compress my lungs well enough for me to breathe. As the months and years passed, I only became more profoundly disabled and my health, precariously fragile.

My journey through the landscape of illness and dysfunction is remarkable in many ways, one being that while my symptoms were seemingly psychogenic, both my physicians and I knew that I was dying. But even as I endured severe weakness and physical dependency, and was classified as a palliative-care patient (i.e., incapable of cure), my suffering and needs were overshadowed by the belief of medical professionals that they were not, in fact, real, and that I was some sort of emotional con artist, intent on exploiting valuable medical resources and attention. The more ill and vulnerable I became, the more I became a medical pariah. I experienced a profound sense of alienation, isolation, and disenfranchisement. My sickness immersed me in not only in the typical suffering that sickness brings but also in a realm in which my very sanity was questioned. Both I and my story were "incredible," not to be believed.[1]

---

1. This clinical "disbelief" of me and my symptoms was documented in a made-for-TV film, *Not Yet Diagnosed* (1997). The film, which is no longer available, depicted my

This climate of disbelief only began to ease once I received a "real" diagnosis. A neurologist once told me (before he dismissed my ailments as psychosomatic) that I had either a "rare manifestation of a common disease or a common manifestation of a rare disease." In the end, it turned out that he wasn't *quite* right, for it seems that some physicians believe that I may have a *rare* presentation of a *rare* disease, myasthenia gravis. At the very least, I respond very well to medications that are usually prescribed for the disease. The literature on MG is rather scant, but the odds of its occurrence are variously estimated to be between one and two cases per million.[2] A factor inhibiting its detection is that it cannot be picked up by X-ray, computed tomography (CT), or magnetic resonance imaging (MRI) scans. Its proper diagnosis depends on a neurological exam, a specific drug test (usually administered by injection or intravenously), specific electrical tests, and blood antibody tests—none of which are considered definitive by themselves (though some experts disagree about even this point). So perhaps it is not surprising that it took so long to accurately categorize my symptoms. Nonetheless, the over ten years of medical fumbling had a devastating effect on me. It had far-reaching physical, emotional, spiritual, financial, social, and political consequences—it disrupted every aspect of my life.

Moreover, as my story reveals, the cause of doctors' disbelief in me is complicated and multivariant. It is the result of a medical culture and hierarchy, and even of a medical architecture, that encourages certain ways of thinking and patterns of behavior. I'd like to think that my experience is unique—and it is, in terms of the depth and severity of my illness, before any proper diagnosis was made and any effective treatment undertaken—but it also isn't. People often leave their doctor's office with a diagnosis of stress-related or psychogenic illness—and, these categories

---

futile efforts to get a "real" diagnosis from a medical specialist. Fortunately, by the end of taping, my family doctor agreed to put me on immune suppressant drugs, which precipitated my recovery (although this was not discussed in the documentary itself).

2. Interestingly, a neurologist who treated me in upstate New York suspected that the incidence of myasthenia gravis was probably more frequent than the official statistics rendered but that the disease was likely misdiagnosed as stress or fatigue (especially in the elderly), and thus patients suffocated to death before being accurately assessed and treated.

do not help patients get better. The existing medical literature reports that at least half of all those who consult doctors manifest symptoms that are psychological in origin and are the result of unresolved emotional stress, and which include headaches, stomach problems, and menstrual cramps. In particular, many medical professionals tend to view young women's physical complaints as emotionally rooted. Research shows that even when men and women have conclusively similar and severe heart disease, male patients are treated more aggressively than female patients. Unfortunately, the psychologizing of illness, especially for women, is an everyday and potentially dangerous occurrence.

Magazine and newspaper articles, as well as books about illness, remind us that emotional stress influences our health. These texts reinforce an underlying cultural assumption that we can meditate, laugh, and epiphanize our way out of sickness. They assure us that we are all capable of healing ourselves through the honing of our mental capacities—a belief that dovetails nicely with the dominant liberal notion that the individual is the ruler of his/her destiny. Since the late nineteenth century, medical capacities have increased exponentially, making it seem that all symptoms are transparent to the medical gaze. Any symptoms that seem implausible or impenetrable thus become suspect. The logic is unassailable. Because medicine can grasp all that it sees, anything that it cannot grasp therefore doesn't exist. Moreover, the lack of clarity must be the patient's fault because the patient is responsible for all things in his/her life. The confluence of a medical culture that is all-knowing and a societal tendency to view the individual as the vessel of all possibility means that it becomes too easy to blame patients for symptoms that are seemingly inexplicable.

This book tells the story of my immersion into illness and into the medical realm of diagnosis and treatment. As I am not only a patient but also a political and legal theorist and scholar, this book interweaves reflective material about the social construction of gender and illness, the practice of medicine, the illness experience, and the social exclusion associated both with the stigma of mental illness and with gross physical impairment.

On one level it tells the story of an illness that I believe was erroneously diagnosed as being psychological in origin for a decade. This mistake cost me dearly in terms of pain and function. It also very nearly killed me. As I battled my ailments, I also battled "to be believed" and, by extension, to access life-saving therapies. Susan Sontag's *Illness as Metaphor* eloquently argues that the psychological portraits associated with diseases are misleading and destructive. My book is an experiential account that validates her argument. It chronicles the experience of being direly ill but encountering disbelief, dismissal, and even hostility in the health-care setting. Even as I became weaker and weaker and more vulnerable and dependent on care, I became increasingly vilified by physicians. In my late twenties, as I lay in intensive care, I heard debates break out around my bedside about whether I was worthy of medical resources and/or medical rescue. For many, the fact that I was so chronically debilitated worked against me; moreover, that the cause of my debility was unknown and therefore presumed to be psychological made me even more grossly contemptible.

But while many physicians remained dubious, there were a remarkable few who always treated me with dignity and who fought to save my life when others dismissed me as unworthy and incurable. It was through their efforts that I was eventually properly diagnosed and treated. My subsequent recovery was quite literally a rebirth in which I moved from total and complete paralysis, requiring ventilator and ICU care, to walking without any assistive aids.

This then is an illness narrative that relates an admixture of suffering, sickness, and being disbelieved, from which I and my family eventually emerge into relative normalcy. Not only does my paralysis recede, but I recover the consciousness that I am not, and never have been, so emotionally unstable as to make myself ill.

At another level, this memoir describes a neurological condition, which, if not myasthenia gravis, is similar to myasthenia gravis and has yet to be portrayed to any extent outside of medical textbooks. Researchers have discovered that MG is an autoimmune disease much like rheumatoid arthritis or multiple sclerosis. Suppressing a patient's immune system can thus result in a reduction in symptoms or even in total remission. As in cases of myasthenia gravis, my own symptoms largely resolved once I received immunosuppressants. What is unique about this condition is that while my illness never totally disappears, with the appropriate management, my symptoms can be suppressed to the point that I can pass as able-bodied. To most observers, I walk, talk, and breathe just like everyone else. To achieve this requires all sorts of medication and careful planning of my schedule. And, unfortunately, I can have a "crisis" that plunges me back into total paralysis. I can require life support and intensive care and, eventually, rehabilitation therapies to recover my breathing, speaking, swallowing, moving, and walking. There is no other ailment that places the patient in this extraordinary paradox of being relatively normal one moment and almost completely "locked-in," that is, aware but unable to communicate because nearly all voluntary muscles are paralyzed, in the next. The pendulum swings very far, but even after a major crisis, with proper medical intervention (as is true of most myasthenics), I return to a condition of relative normalcy.

At a third level, this story gives voice to a rare and singular experience of extreme physical vulnerability and disability—a condition that is usually experienced by those near death or who are so severely and totally physically or mentally handicapped that they never fully recover and thus remain unable to communicate with others. My experience is one that is usually characterized by silence as it is the result of a physical condition that, most often, can only be observed and talked about from the outside and thus only at a superficial level. Neurologists have little knowledge of what types of consciousness exist in patients who are totally paralyzed. Without the means to communicate or move, many such patients are presumed to be lacking in brain function. Breakthroughs in electrical scans of the brain during the early part of this century have resulted in clinicians realizing that nonresponsive patients have more awareness than first conjectured. This, then, is an account from the "inside"—it is the view from within a state of extraordinary physical helplessness and incapacity.[3]

---

3. Jean Dominique Bauby's *The Diving Bell and the Butterfly: A Memoir of Life in Death* (*Le scaphandre et le papillion*) stands as an example of a similar type of account. Bauby,

But, finally, and perhaps most important, this book is a political document—it is a justice narrative. This work chronicles the deliberate, and sometimes aggressive, refusal of physicians to aid and treat an acutely ill and vulnerable patient. Even though the patient is fully insured and mentally competent, she is consistently disbelieved and her symptoms are dismissed as illegitimate. It is only through the utmost stubborn conviction that her own symptoms are real, along with the actions of a few select and extraordinary clinicians, that the patient is eventually rescued.

This book illustrates that medicine's belief in evidence-based practice does not mean that it is devoid of prejudicial views and behaviors that can greatly impair its seeming objectivity. In fact, evidence-based medicine can reinforce clinical and cultural stereotypes because it does not take into account those symptoms and cases that fall outside statistical norms. Moreover, as both medical schools and hospitals have tried to take a more humane and holistic approaches to patients—due, in large part, to illness narratives itemizing the gross insensitivities of the medical establishment—these efforts have not necessarily yielded their intended results. My story demonstrates the multiplicity of factors that lead to a psychogenic diagnosis and it explores the malleability and imprecision of such diagnoses and the dangers that all patients face in a medical world in which psychological profiling of disease is increasingly commonplace. On the surface such profiling is part of medicine's aim to become more holistic—to treat the patient more wholly, taking into account his or her mind, body, and soul—however, despite this admirable goal, it can, at minimum, lead to an individual feeling responsible for his or her illness, or maximally, lead to a patient being vilified and "psychiatrized" for not getting well. While clinicians speak of treating the person as whole, from the patient's perspective, medicine seems only to respond as though one is either mentally ill *or* physically ill. As such, the clinical

---

former editor of *Elle* magazine, suffered a massive stroke that left him with locked-in syndrome. He could communicate only by blinking one eye. An assistant verbally worked her way through a frequency alphabet, and Bauby blinked at the correct letter, painstakingly spelling out his memoir. He died two days after its original publication in 1997. A film version of this memoir was released in early 2008.

disciplines, medical subspecialties, nursing, and even the very design of hospital wards reinforce a compartmentalized view of the human being. When ambiguous physical symptoms are presumed to be psychological in origin by default, patients find themselves confined within calcified psychological stereotypes (and sometimes psychiatric wards) that result in treatment that is far from holistic and that does not effectively encompass the extraordinary and incalculable interpenetration of the mind and body.

This book, thus, chronicles a physical journey while simultaneously elucidating our culture's problematic understanding of sickness. Liberal democracies evoke a paradigm of equal, autonomous, and fit citizenship. To require care challenges this paradigm. To ail physically means confronting one's dependence in a society that eagerly extols individual autonomy and independence. Psychological theories of disease reflect this ethos by positing that sick individuals somehow incite, determine, and shape their illnesses. Picking up where Susan Sontag leaves off in *Illness as Metaphor,* in this book I attack the prevailing norm that certain types of people become ill with certain types of diseases. The book clearly delineates the enormous self-doubt that this assumption creates in patients as well as the highly destructive and even dangerous effect that it can have on patients' medical care. It also shows how easily medical professionals reach for psychological theories of sickness when they are confronted by symptoms they do not fully understand—how difficult it is for them to say, "I don't know, let's try to find out together," and how easy it is for them to start blaming the patient. As such, this is a substantive critique of the psychologizing of disease (to which we are all subject as patients) and of medical certainty in the face of ambiguous human morbidity and mortality. I draw on an array of scholarly and medical literature with which to clarify and analyze my overall narrative. My observations as a political and legal theorist are never far from those I make as a patient. I assess medical culture, education, and architecture as well as the practice of biomedical ethics from within the garb of being ill and of being treated within modern health-care settings. Theories and criticism thus interpenetrate the chronicle of patienthood.

But while this book challenges the destructive disbeliefs that result from an unassailable medical system that is often unable to accept illnesses and symptoms that are not easily diagnosed or known, it also recognizes the incredible capacities of modern medical technologies and practices. I know that my survival is both *in spite of* medical treatment and *because of* it. The resuscitations, the intubations, ventilators, and plasmapheresis procedures are all the result of a technocratic medicine of which I am critical but that has also kept me alive. Moreover, the drug therapies that now allow me a relatively normal existence and have allowed me to produce a burgeoning family are all the result of medical innovations in the past two decades. Quite simply, if I had been born in another place, in another time, I would not be alive, let alone be an academic, a spouse, and a parent. Paradoxically, while medicine, in its disbelief in me, inflicted a bizarre form of suffering for over a decade, it also rescued, and continues to rescue, me with an array of complex and sometimes toxic drug therapies. For this second life, I am immeasurably grateful.

I turned forty this year, a birthday that I never thought I would make. When I was in my early twenties, my godfather, a rather eccentric physician who lived in the Lake District in England, made an ominous prediction. We stood on a rise behind his house. I was leaning on a cane and struggling to breath in the damp early spring air. "You will not live to make forty," he said. Others provided even more dire forecasts. Now, I look back in awe that I actually made it through both the abyss of my illness and the medical treatment that accompanied it.

The fact that we finally arrived at a physical cause, diagnosis, and treatment for my illness is the result of an admixture of my own pigheadedness; the devout caring of my spouse, children, and friends; and the support and tenacity of a minority of clinicians, who, despite prevailing evidence—or nonevidence—and opinion, always treated me with respect and continued to ponder the possibility that my illness was, indeed, "real." It is thus only through stubbornness and good fortune that I managed to access life-saving technologies and medicines.

It amazes me that the human body has the strength to return from total immobility to relative able-bodiedness in the way that mine has.

In his autobiography, Christopher Nolan writes that the ghosts of silent and mute crippled men haunt him as he writes. Nolan has cerebral palsy and has limited voluntary movement in his neck. He does not speak but has found a voice through tapping out prose on a keyboard with a unicorn stick attached to his head. After years of debility and shame, I, too, sense the mute energy of those who never return from such deep agony and vulnerable paralyses. I was lucky: an ambiguous grace reached down and released me from my torment. I write this book for those who never receive such amnesty, whether because they die or because they remain bound by uncooperative muscles. I also write for the many more who experience, or will experience, curious and inexplicable symptoms for which doctors can find no cause.

In the end, medicine wields extraordinary powers that can be constructive and/or destructive. Perhaps we can become more aware of the ambivalence of all illnesses and of the type of doubt that ambiguity evokes in clinical staff. For it is at these moments that clinicians can act blindly and reflexively—wounding instead of healing.

It is my hope that this account of my long and ongoing struggle with a disease deemed imaginary and of the clinicians who stood in the way of my recovery challenges the dangers of an unassailable medical system and provokes a major shift in the way we think about, treat, and define conditions that often defy categorization.

My Imaginary Illness

1 *Beginnings*

In the spring of 1986, I was twenty years old and finishing my last year of undergraduate education at the University of Toronto. I was much younger than my peers, having entered university when I was two years younger than most Ontario college students (who, at the time, completed thirteen years of school before entering college). I was thus used to being "ahead" of everyone else. But for the first time in my life, I had fallen behind. I left campus without completing my honors senior thesis. I had had to undergo major abdominal surgery for an ovarian cyst in January and took a month's hiatus from schoolwork. I had scrambled to catch up with my studies during the final weeks of the term. In the end, I simply lacked the time and energy to complete my project.

Consequently, as I packed up my dorm room, my intention was to go tree planting in northern British Columbia for ten weeks to earn a cache of money, visit Expo in Vancouver, and then return to Toronto to complete my paper sometime during the late summer and early fall. After handing in my thesis, I imagined that I would then apply to graduate school in English or political science or law school or medical school and then set off on a trek across Europe or Asia as I awaited various universities' decisions. While I did not have an "A" average, all of my grades were either in the "A" or "B+" range, and I presumed that this type of academic performance, accompanied by my membership on two varsity sports teams in rowing and squash, my election to my college board of regents, my participation in the university's select writing seminar, my part-time jobs, and my strong standardized tests scores (i.e., the GRE and LSAT) would create a good impression with admissions committees.

In short, I was confident that my future held promise. Unfortunately, I was wrong.

My fantasies tended to downplay a few disturbing things that I was experiencing. First, I seemed irrevocably estranged from my parents and brother. But, more important, during the past two years I had begun to experience strange physical sensations that I dismissed as either my "getting old" or as my becoming morally "weak." For example, during my sophomore year, I found myself unusually fatigued and was diagnosed by the health center staff with mononucleosis. I didn't have a fever during this period, and, while I usually felt renewed after lying down, the ongoing sense of being exhausted never really left me. Over the next twenty-four months I found myself having prolonged feelings of fatigue and needing to lie down more often. The lethargy and vague ill feeling would disappear for a few weeks only to return again and again. My general practitioner (GP) suggested that as I still tested positive for the Epstein-Barr virus I simply had a lengthy form of the illness. I remained unsure but did my best to ignore my symptoms.

Yet, during this period, I also suddenly lost my ability to throw a ball with any accuracy. My undergraduate college held pickup games of soccer and stickball in the field between the dorms. Among my friends I'd gained a reputation for being an evil stickball pitcher. (As a child, my favorite stroke in tennis had been the serve, and I discovered that the two motions of pitching and serving were very similar.) But one evening my throwing was ludicrously poor. The ball bounced ten feet in front of the batter or flew yards to either side. The players laughed at first, but after I made several tries, they grew impatient. Embarrassed by my clumsiness, I withdrew from the field mumbling something about getting old. I had no idea what had happened. A week or so later, I tried again. The first couple of pitches seemed better, but once again my accuracy and speed collapsed. I stopped playing stickball.

I also felt uneasy when I played other sports. Some days, practice with the squash team roared along. But on others, I couldn't seem to follow my coach's instructions to alter my stroke or stance. My body seemed disconnected and sluggish. More and more, I found myself tripping as I ran uphill or upstairs. I assumed that I was simply not paying close enough attention, that I needed to increase my focus and effort. In addition, muscles in my face and shoulders would sometimes twitch minutely and involuntarily for days.

But, as I packed my duffel bag to head out west to the forests of British Columbia, I didn't make much of these incidents. They were not really part of my consciousness nor did they form any part of my sense of myself and of my capacities. (It is only now, years later and with the benefit of hindsight that I wonder whether these were ominous hints of my future troubles.)

A day or so later I stood in the parking lot of a motel in Prince George, British Columbia, with a yellow duffel bag slumped at my feet and a sleeping bag tucked under my arm, waiting to share a ride to the "plantation"—that is, the worksite for planting trees. I had spent the previous night trying to sleep in Edmonton International Airport in Alberta as cleaners rumbled interminable trains of luggage carts back and forth across the tiled floor. Standing and breathing in the acrid air of the pulp paper town, I felt tired and unwell. A migraine pounded down one side of my head, and I felt nauseated.

Eventually, a filthy pale blue pickup truck pulled into the driveway, and an equally dirty, but effervescent, blond-haired young man leaned out the window and greeted me. The driver introduced himself with a broad smile and extended a deeply creased, grubby hand. "Jim," he simply said. "You must be Chloë, right? I came for you yesterday, but then I realized I got the day wrong." He stroked his reddish, stubbly chin, "Like the beard, eh?" and then laughed good-naturedly. His eyes shone brightly amid his unkempt hair and face. "I'm your boss for the next two months." He looked at me as I shifted my weight awkwardly from foot to foot, waiting for instructions. "Well, let's get goin'." He gestured behind him, "Put your stuff back there and hop in. We got a three-hour drive ahead of us."

My bags fell amid orange fuel containers, tangled ropes, chainsaws, metal tool chests, and mud-smeared ice coolers in the bed of the truck. The cab had receipts jammed into the glove compartment, and used coffee cups and beer bottles rolled about on the floor. "You eaten?" he asked.

"A bit."

"Let's grab a burger on the way."

"Sure."

Soon the smell of chemical cheese and grease filled my nostrils as I propped myself up against the passenger door and allowed the growl and vibration of the engine to overtake me. The pain in my head gradually dissipated as I meditated myself into a state of semiconsciousness.

I spent the next few days crawling around the plantation on my hands and knees. Our camp lay against a steep mountainside amid a moonscape of deforestation. The snow-covered peaks seemed to be the only untouched portion of the landscape. Huge uprooted tree trunks and deciduous saplings required arduous climbing around and ducking under as I tried to plant each tree plug. It was rare to be able to take two unhampered steps. Tree bags hung from harnesses across my shoulders and I wore a belt around my hips. I held a shovel in one hand and my other hand was encased in a cold, sodden cotton-silicon glove. Within hours, broken blisters oozed on my palms and between my fingers and toes.

At night frost formed on the outer layer of my sleeping bag. During the day, it either snowed or hailed or the sun shone with a relentless intensity. It seemed that the climate was never benevolent, but it was more the isolated, brutal nature of the work that made the weather seem so inclement.

The number of trees planted determined my wage. Depending on the terrain, a single tree plug (properly spaced and secured in mineral soil) was worth anywhere from ten to twenty-five cents. Experienced, high-rolling planters earned over a hundred dollars a day (a large sum in those days). During my first week I was lucky if I made forty. Some days, after I deducted my costs, I made nothing. But gradually, my speed, my skills, and thus my earnings improved. It seemed as though I might not only survive the ordeal but perhaps also emerge with a bit of money.

The austere landscape and hard physical labor were captivating, but not enough to mask a sharp ache in my abdomen that interrupted my work, my reveries, and even my sleep. I began to wonder whether the solid ovarian cyst I had removed the previous winter had somehow reoccurred. While the crew's faces were creased with exhaustion, I wondered whether my persistent sense of stumbling fatigue was uniquely my own or was to be overlooked as part of the job. At a vague level, my body did not feel my own; at a specific level, I felt a jabbing pain. On a trip to town to fill up on gas, cigarettes, groceries, and tree boxes, I visited the local clinic. After performing an ultrasound, the ob-gyn suggested that I needed abdominal laparoscopic surgery. He assured me that he could snip out what ailed me with little or no invasive cutting or suturing. I hesitated. My previous (and only) operation had been a "full abdominal": The surgeons had laid my organs on my chest and had gone through them piecemeal to ensure that none of the tumor had been left behind. The surgical resident confessed that I had been long to rouse and hard to wean from the ventilator. My own recollection was of feeling as though I had been run over by a streetcar. I was suspicious of the gynecologist's assurances but knew that I needed to do something. I also suspected that my anxieties were likely overwrought—I worried too much. Of course, I thought to myself, he was right; I'd be on my feet and out of the hospital within twenty-four hours. I signed the consent form.

2 The Original Crisis

The first thing I remember is not being able to see. My eyes were open; at least it felt that way. But I couldn't be sure because I'd just woken up. My eyes shifted heavily. I shut them and waited a little. A voice urged me, "Dear, it's time to wake up now!" I opened my lids again and saw only opaque shadows moving above me. "Wake up, dear! Wake up!...What's her name?!" I heard my name over and over, sometimes gentle, sometimes insistent: "Open your eyes!"

Jesus, I thought, my eyes are open. And then I realized I couldn't see clearly. The world was underwater—blurred and unfocused. And then I felt hands laid on indistinct parts of my body. "Hhhaa!" I called out, my tongue lolling heavily. "Aaaah cann nn seee." My tongue labored in the cavern of my mouth. Hands deftly bound my body with sheets and slung me through the air onto another stretcher. I felt the hiss of oxygen on my face.

Some time later, a male voice persisted through the gloom, "Squeeze my fingers."

I squeezed his index and middle fingers.

"Squeeze them!"

What? Squeeze them? I just squeezed them! The fingers of my right hand reached out, groping for his hand. They searched the blanket and lunged at the dark shape in front of me.

"No. No, with the other hand. Your left hand. Squeeze with your left hand!"

My left hand....Where was my left hand? Finally, I felt his hand in mine. Thank god. I squeezed with all my strength.

"Now I want you to do it harder than that. Do it harder!"

At the same time, I wanted to yell, "Not my hand, you idiot! My eyes! I can't see. It's my eyes!" I grasped his fingers while simultaneously trying to twist my body away from his vociferous authority.

"Okay. Sit up!" His dark form hung over me.

I threw my head forward, but my chin rolled to one side and my chest sagged leadenly against the mattress. Shit, I thought. I grabbed at the bed rail with one hand and pulled. I slid awkwardly onto my right elbow.

"Sit up!"

I tried again, but my torso rolled softly away. A man's forearm gathered me at the shoulders and drew me into a sitting position.

"Raise your left arm....*Raise* your left arm!"

I felt something cool and dead fish–like lying on my right thigh. I pushed it away.

"Don't use your other arm, raise it yourself!"

Desperately, I reasoned to myself, "Other arm? Other arm. Yes. Two arms. I have two arms." I knew that I should know that I had two arms. I should have seen and felt them. But all I could do was panic.

A warm palm touched me. I felt the pad of the man's thumb against my wrist. He lifted the arm in front of me. I could feel it. "That's right. That's right. Hold it higher....Try again, hold it up....Now shut your eyes and keep it there."

With my eyes closed it disappeared.

"Okay now, you can open them."

I looked, but the shadow-arm-thing wasn't there. The thing, my arm, was down by my leg, near the sheet.

"Okay." He straightened up. "Oh yeah, I'm Dr. A. I'll be looking after you." He patted the bed with his notebook as he turned to leave. "I'll see you later."

A few hours later more physicians arrived. Without introduction, they stood around my bed, the sheets pulled back, my supine body laid before them. Again insistent voices asked me to move, sit, see, feel, speak.

The uncooperative oddity of my body embarrassed and frightened me. My body had lost grace—a grace and power that, at the age of twenty, I had presumed I would always have. And now I lay like a sandbag, fighting the weight of inertia that seemed to encase my limbs. I desperately wanted to believe nothing was wrong.

But, after several days, I still lay in the same postsurgical ward room by the window. Women occupied the other beds intermittently, most staying no more than a couple of nights. My eyesight improved: the blurriness eased, but I couldn't see fine detail. A tattered paperback copy of Conrad's *Lord Jim* that I had taken with me into "the bush" a few weeks earlier lay unread on the window sill.

With my stronger right arm I could grab the opposite bed rail and roll onto my weak left side. I pulled and pushed myself from back to side, side to back, back to side, searching for comfort on top of the plastic-covered mattress. Internally, I felt a deep, tearing pain, as though my hip bone was impaling my flesh. My fidgeting seemed to rotate my torso around a single portion of bone and skin.

Through the window, I stared at brilliant skies and breathed the town's polluted air. My body would gradually slip lower and lower in the bed. Once in a while, a nurse would come to straighten my sheets and pull my body back up to the top of the mattress. Finally, one of them turned to me and said, "You can call us to move you." She pointed at the cable and bell pinned to my gown, "That's what this is for." Dumbfounded, I smiled to thank her. Although my tongue no longer rolled thickly in my mouth, I couldn't bring myself to ask for help for something as apparently simple as rolling over in bed.

Imbued with a stoic attitude and a stubborn sense of self-reliance that had seen me through boarding school, university, and a deteriorating relationship with my parents, I lacked the psychological capacity to grasp my utter dependency. Even when one middle-aged woman who was being wheeled off for day surgery gestured at me and said fiercely, "I don't want to end up like her!" I continued to deny the extent and depth of my vulnerability.

One evening, about two weeks after I first awoke, five physicians gathered around my bed to discuss my case. The overall consensus was that I had had a stroke during laparoscopic surgery twelve days before. Disagreement arose over its cause and my prognosis. The first CT scan read as negative, the second showed some sort of abnormality in the right cerebral hemisphere, but its significance remained ambiguous. As they debated various medical possibilities while standing in a semicircle, I felt myself foundering.

Just minutes earlier, two nurses had treated my dormant bowels with an enema. They had rolled up the head of the bed and propped me unceremoniously on top of a bedpan. As the medical staff rounded the curtain, they had yanked up the bedsheets as camouflage. My body was now erupting uncontrollably beneath me as I tried to hold on to the tendrils of conversation. I felt supremely debased by the spectacle of myself defecating in front of an assembly and simultaneously hoped and feared that the stench would soon drive people from the room. But they stood steadfast: two surgeons, an anesthesiologist, a consulting neurologist, and a physiatrist (rehabilitation specialist) each presented his or her theory to me. Although, I felt my vision dim and my breath labor, the physicians politely carried on. Finally, after a seemingly interminable presentation, they left my bedside with a gentle flapping of the privacy curtain. The last one, a young surgeon, patted my arm reassuringly and said, "Don't worry, you'll get better."

Almost immediately, the two nurses swept in. "Gosh, we're sorry to have left you for so long," they laughed. "We didn't know they'd stay!"

They pulled back the covers to reveal my spasming body and an excretory mess. "Oooo, I think we need help."

One turned to the other, "Joanie, get Barb and Simon in here right away!"

Within moments, deft arms heaved me off the bed. The assistants ducked under IV lines to tear away soiled gowns and bed clothes. As my body continued to involuntarily leak fluids, solid arms lifted me toward the temporary refuge of a clean stretcher. But in midair, a wave of nausea overtook me. My stomach began to heave. The nurses' uniforms, the floor, and lights merged and swirled incomprehensibly as I passed out.

I awoke with an oxygen mask hissing damply on my face and the young surgeon leaning obscurely over me, asking, "What happened? Your saturations dropped through the floor."[1]

I knew full well what had happened but could only mumble, "I don't know." I didn't know how to explain that the mere act of defecating had defeated me.

More than that I wanted to know what was wrong with me. I was only twenty, and I'd lain there for two weeks and no one seemed to know what was wrong.

And I hated—always had hated—being sick ever since I was a child. The helplessness of illness unnerved me. I can remember hiding under the bed when the pediatrician made house calls. He would lift up the bedcovers and peer in at me, coaxing me to come out. I felt far too naked in my nightgown to be in his presence. I also knew that despite his seeming benevolence, his instruments always hurt my ears. When I was a bit older, on mornings when I lay in bed too long, I castigated myself. Lying in bed or remaining in pajamas felt reprobate, not necessarily because it indicated slothfulness but because I associated it with the shame of being unproductively sick.

And here I was immobile on the surgical ward. While I began to understand that I needed help, I tried to maintain a facade of cheer and bravado. I did not want to be self-pitying. Likewise, I feared that any demonstration of anger or despair would make me unlikable in the eyes of those who cared for me. I felt dependent on my caregivers' goodwill and thus found myself involuntarily courting nurses' and doctors' favor with smiles and gratitude. I couldn't stop myself. Unconsciously, I intuited that my care, while in the hospital, was imbedded in an inchoate matrix of power.

---

1. Oxygen saturation denotes the amount of oxygen that the blood haemoglobin carries. It is measured through the skin by a sensor placed on the earlobe or fingertip. Normal oxygen saturations run between 92 and 98 percent.

What I did not know at the time was that the severity of my symptoms, as well as the indeterminacy of signs and tests, meant that my doctors were considering that I might have a hysterical illness—in other words, that my weakness and paralysis might be the result of my psyche and not the product of an "organic" process. In medical terms, they were considering what is called a "functional" or psychosomatic illness. I would not know this for several weeks. Nonetheless, I sensed a hesitancy on the part of some staff members with regard to their demeanor that made me even more uneasy.

When the neurologist and other treating physicians seemed puzzled by what had happened to me, I should have worried. They supposed, they told me, that I had "had a stroke—but that the evidence, so far, is not definitive." What I did not know was that the field of medicine does not tolerate uncertainty very well. Medical personnel are trained to reach a diagnosis. And an array of equipment and laboratory tests exist to facilitate their efforts. Within the allopathic medical model, once a patient has a diagnostic label, appropriate interventions, treatments, and plans can be made. Symptoms, even severe ones such as paralysis and difficulty breathing, are meaningless if they fail to fit into set diagnostic criteria. Thus, unbeknown to me, I was not only physically vulnerable, I was increasingly in jeopardy because no one knew why I was sick. There seemed to be only three choices. One, I could be suffering from an as yet undiagnosed rare illness. Two, my physicians were incompetent. Three, my symptoms were stress induced (i.e., they were psychological) in origin. None of these possibilities was very attractive.

3 *Facing Uncertainty*

Clinicians often turn to psychosomatic diagnoses when they can find no organic cause for an individual's complaints. Patients who have symptoms that do not fit into well-understood physiological patterns easily fall under the rubric of "not yet diagnosed" (NYD) and/or somatoform or hysterical disorders. In this sense, they challenge received notions of what it is, in fact, to be "diseased." Hysterical symptoms are ones that do not fit comfortably within traditional medical conceptions and classifications. They introduce uncertainty into the process of diagnosis. While subjectively the symptoms remain very real for the sufferer, objectively they offer no clinical evidence for their existence. As a result, psychosomatic diagnoses exist in an ambiguous conceptual realm—lying somewhere between the boundaries of the physical, mental, spiritual, and cultural spheres of human existence. They are diagnoses of ambiguity. Controversy and discomfort often characterize this type of diagnosis.

Historically, the medical nosology for diagnostic cataloging finds its origins in botanical and biological systems of classification. The main purpose of having a diagnosis is to provide groupings of symptoms and phenomena that are efficacious in choosing a medical treatment. Diseases, then, are not concrete entities, but are conceptual models that are used to try to combat sickness and prolong human life. As a popular health writer points out: "Disease classifications are even further removed from concrete objects than animal or plant classifications. At least an individual oak tree being classified is a tangible 'thing'" (Ziporyn 1992, 88).

The abstract modeling of disease constantly shifts and changes. Through the centuries, medicine has employed a variety of frameworks with which to understand the human body and its illnesses. Humoral systems of medical knowledge produce different disease categories than do paradigms of germ theory or more technologically based models. Moreover, in modern medicine, different subspecialties often comprehend diseases differently. For instance, immunological medical theory is quite different from rehabilitative medical theory. Definitions of disease thus change according to the context in which they are formed and employed.

Determining whether a patient has a disease type that can be treated requires that the clinician interpret symptomatology that is the result not only of diagnostic definitions but also of moral, cultural, familial, and personal value systems.

As such, the philosopher Ian Hacking argues that disease classifications do not solidify unless they fit a specific social context (Hacking 1998). The stability of disease typing provides tremendous benefit to both the ill individual and the physician. Medicine's use of categories simplifies diverse bodily signs into interpretable symptoms. This simplification has a fundamental power in its capacity to treat illness. It codifies symptoms so that they can be potentially treated and ameliorated. Plans can be made and courses of action taken. Hopes and fears are focused on a tangible entity. Together the patient and practitioner attempt to resolve the amorphous void of illness and replace it with the clearer certainty of disease. In this sense, they both dislike ambivalence. They desire solutions to what may be bewildering and overwhelming problems—and disease categories provide such solutions. Practitioners and patients thus form a symbiotic relationship in which the meaning and significance of a disease can be easily understood and accepted by both parties.

There are a number of weaknesses in this dynamic, however. First, in forcing certitude on ambiguous and unfathomable situations, diagnoses can coerce complex human beings into simplified paradigms. In her writings on tuberculosis, cancer, and AIDS, the late cultural critic Susan

Sontag proposed that diseases become metaphors that tend to characterize individual patients. These can harden to the extent that they come to dominate the patient's medical persona. Second, this reification is particularly true in the realm of psychological illnesses. Psychological theories of illness can be easily flexed to fit a wide range of signs and symptoms. Feminist theorist Kate Millett, in writing about her own experience of mental illness, observes that "diagnosis is based upon impressionistic evidence: conduct, deportment, and social manner. Such evidence is frequently misinterpreted" (Millett 1990, 311). The diagnosis of a mental disorder, over a physical one, can cause even greater injury. Mental diseases—of which psychogenic/hysterical disorders are a marginal part—carry enormous stigma. As theories of psychological abnormality, they easily create self-doubt and social ostracism for the patient. Third, diagnostic categories define eligibility for health and life insurance. They arbitrate not only whether someone will receive treatment but that person's access to pharmaceuticals and other remedies. Fourth and finally, diagnoses (and especially mental health diagnoses) define what type of sick role an individual can adopt within her social community—that is, whether she is legitimately ill or not and whether she is thereby deserving of social supports.

In the beginning, as I confronted my weakness and paralysis, I had no sense of this dynamic. I viewed medicine much the way television dramas (and popular culture) presented it: as a highly technological field with an all-knowing capacity to diagnose, treat, and cure illness.

It only gradually occurred to me that the trajectory of my own sickness was not adhering to popular projections. I began to realize that a person can easily be branded with a particular diagnosis that, like a scarlet letter, follows the patient and shapes her medical fate—sometimes so rigidly that facts and data that contradict that diagnosis are summarily dismissed and denied.

Unfortunately, I would be involved in this process for the next twelve years.

4 Ontological Apprehensions

Weeks dragged by in the hospital in northern British Columbia as I awaited transfer to a facility across the country in Toronto. When I awoke each morning, I would try to guess what position my limbs were laying in; I found it astonishing that I often couldn't tell where they lay without looking at them. Paradoxically, I found that my weaker hand felt surfaces and temperatures in astonishing detail. Water felt hotter and colder than it did with my stronger hand. Smooth surfaces undulated with ridges that were usually imperceptible. These novel sensations both intrigued and terrified me. I sensed that I was having an ontological crisis: I no longer knew who I was and what was real. If one hand gave me one set of perceptions about the world and the other hand gave me an entirely different set, which was truer? If a physical injury to the nervous system or brain could so easily fracture my understanding of the material world, what then was reality? And more important, what was my true self? The self that perceived the wash water to be quite hot? Or the self that felt it to be only tepid? What, also, was the relationship of the will to the self? I had always seen myself as a strong-willed person, but what if my will wasn't anything more than a biochemical process that could be destroyed or damaged by a physical illness? The admiration that society expresses for those who overcome disability and physical hardship might simply be misguided. Will might simply be a matter of luck rather than character;

will as a biological fact that either remains intact or is destroyed by disease might be the difference between the patient who lives and recovers versus the one who dies or remains crippled. The hospital staff kept reiterating that I needed to remain "positive" and fight against this bizarre illness, but who was "I" really? The "I" who knew the metal bed frame was smooth? Or the "I" who felt it to be microscopically ridged? The self I had relied on so deeply to push myself through challenges now confronted seemingly irreconcilable inputs. How could I know that my outputs would be stable—that I would be the same old self who faced down obstacles with stubborn and irritating insistence?

These questions persisted as I made inconsistent gains. One day I would be able to move my leg a certain way and the next day I wouldn't. Some days I could sit up in a wheelchair for a couple of hours, other days I passed out. The physiotherapist and doctors were kind, but they scolded me for my seemingly uneven effort. I became embarrassed and frustrated by my ineptitude. The doctors often told me that stroke patients recovered differently than I seemed to be doing. They gently reprimanded me with phrases such as "CVAs don't move that way"[1] or "Your reflexes seem to vary slightly every day" or "You could move that muscle yesterday." As a result, the medical staff treated me with benevolent but puzzled concern.

The absence of my immediate family made matters worse. My paternal grandfather had been a renowned breast cancer surgeon. (He had died a few years earlier when I was seventeen.) He was the first professor of surgery at Guy's Hospital in London; he had been president of the Royal College of Physicians and Surgeons and had been knighted twice for his medical service. My parents themselves were well-off and well-connected Canadians. Given my family's medical and social standing, the staff could not understand why my parents had abandoned me. Was there a substantial reason? My parents' absence made me suspect. To complicate matters, one of my physicians had trained under my grandfather during his medical schooling in England. This only enhanced his wariness of me, for he

---

1. CVA stands for "cerebral vascular accident," another term for stroke.

could not imagine the family of his old mentor abandoning a relative. My physicians thus treated me with a bewildered kindness that masked scepticism about my psychological and social stability.

The American Academy of Family Physicians defines a family as a group of "individuals with continuing legal, genetic and/or emotional relationships. The family is expected by society to provide for the economic and protective needs of its members particularly children and the elderly" (Mravcak 2006, 280). Physicians and other health-care providers reasonably presume and expect that families will be involved in patients' illnesses and consequent medical care. This is particularly true when children, young adults, and/or the elderly become ill. It is now common for children's hospitals to encourage parents to stay overnight with their ailing sons or daughters. Bedside couches or benches convert easily into single beds for the attending parent. Adult hospitals have also begun to do the same. The University of Maryland Medical Center's new intensive surgical care unit for adults has been designed to facilitate family members staying overnight.[2] Increasingly, hospitals and other health-care facilities provide comfortable accommodations for patients' family members, permitting and encouraging them to spend time at their loved one's bedside, and even staying with them overnight. It is generally assumed that families should, and will want to, be in close contact with their sick family members. Unfortunately, my parents and I simply did not fit this paradigm.

And, so, when I first lay immobilized, the medical practitioners who cared for me wondered why my parents did not immediately fly to my bedside. While I felt lonely without my parents, I had no expectation that they would rescue or care for me. We had not really lived with one another since I had left for boarding school at the age of thirteen, and by the time

---

2. "Waiting rooms in many new facilities now include sleeping accommodations, lockers, private phone and internet booths, playrooms for children, kitchen and pantry facilities, soothing music, and even fish tanks, water falls and nature views. In some cases, overnight stays in the ICU room are encouraged, particularly in pediatric facilities. Many designers now allocate a zone within the ICU room for this purpose. At the Woodwinds Health Campus in St. Paul, for example, the zone closest to the window is the family's domain and can include a sleeper sofa. A similar arrangement is used at Clarian Methodist Hospital in Indianapolis" (Stark 2004, 32).

I became ill at twenty I was legally an adult. Still, my parents' conspicuous absence was not something that was easily explained to the doctors and nurses who gently probed me about my relations with them. This situation appeared to claim the foreground of my caregivers' attention, to preoccupy and perplex them. (A number of years later a psychiatrist involved in my care would remark, "Even murderers' families come to visit them in prison!...What did you do to them?")

In my own case, precisely because clinicians projected their own "family values" onto my quite different family situation, I suffered in their esteem of me. It did not matter that my friends and acquaintances were so effusive in their support for me, that innumerable flower arrangements began to appear by my bed. The windowsill and tables became so full that vases migrated out to the nurse's station and to other patients on the ward. Even my parents' friends—people with whom I had had only sporadic contact for the last few years—called me, sent me telegrams, and mailed me cards and small packages. None of this outpouring of support seemed to counteract the subtle sense of personal deficiency that had been assigned to me as result of my parents' continued absence.

Despite their misgivings, the medical staff devoted a great deal of time and resources to my care. They sought a place for me in a rehabilitation hospital. They wanted to move me to a facility that could provide better diagnostic and therapeutic resources. They explored a variety of options and decided that, even if my parents remained uninvolved in my care, it would be better that I return to a city where I had friends. The hospital approached a local businessman for help, and he offered to fly me across the country in his private jet. Within a week, an ambulance crew loaded me on a stretcher and into a small plane. Later the same day, another ambulance crew greeted me when the jet landed.

Against my wishes, the hospital had informed my parents of the time and place of my arrival. The accompanying nurse chatted expectantly about meeting them, making me vibrate with worry and anticipation. But they didn't meet the plane, nor did they appear when I was admitted to the receiving hospital. The clinical staff who accompanied me could barely disguise their disapproval.

5 Diagnosis: Conversion Reaction

When I got back to Toronto, I became acutely aware of my losses. I measured myself against recent memories of myself walking, training, studying, and working in the familiar cityscape. I felt deeply humiliated. Only weeks before I had bragged to my friends of the small fortune I would make tree planting, about how this money would be used to travel the world or attend graduate or law school. Now I couldn't even work and I was deeply afraid.

One of the first rules I learned as I child was not to show fear. I thus approached the medical staff in the new hospital with a good-natured bravado. I not only wanted but needed them to like me. I realized much later that because somatizing or hysterical patients are meant to demonstrate an inappropriate indifference to their symptomology—*la belle indifference*—my jovial presentation could only have abetted the rising suspicion that my ailments were psychological in origin rather than purely physical.

Clinicians remained circumspect in their dealings with me. They told me little except that they doubted the veracity of the report of the CT scan findings of a few weeks earlier that indicated a "perfusion" in the right hemisphere of my brain. Although the neurology staff physician and senior resident both examined me, when I questioned them, they never spoke to me about a diagnosis and/or plan of treatment. They simply patted my leg and told me I would get better, that I just had to try harder. I did, however, see a physiotherapist and occupational therapist every day. And while I worked arduously at regaining my strength and learning to walk, I never quite managed to eliminate the weakness that affected one side of my body and my core muscles. In addition, I was utterly exhausted. Again, the nurses and therapists chided me for my seeming uneven effort.

I began to get intense migraines from the stress of appearing congenial while feeling completely helpless, silenced, terrified, and alone. I knew I was somatizing my emotional strain, but I couldn't stop myself. And again, my need for pain medications to ease my increasingly frequent migraines probably only fuelled the burgeoning notion that my complaints were intrinsically psychological.

Without warning, a psychiatrist showed up one day. He introduced himself as Dr. C. and asked me to follow him down the hall for an interview. The sense of being ambushed was overwhelming. I immediately knew that he wasn't there to offer support but was instead there on a reconnaissance mission to determine the extent of my emotional disequilibrium. He seemed oblivious to the difficulty that I had in standing and walking and questioned whether it was really necessary for me to use a cane. I remember little of our interview except that he suddenly asked me what I fantasized about during sexual intercourse. This question stunned me. I was a young adult and sexually inexperienced and totally unprepared to discuss such intimacies with a stranger. I wanted to scream that my main concern was whether I would ever walk again. Nonetheless, I answered his query, suspecting that if I refused, I'd give people further proof of my "mental illness." Nonetheless, after a few more similarly phrased questions that made me feel violated and misunderstood, I terminated the interview.

The hospital staff rebuked me for not making better gains. A social worker was assigned to my case, and we met a couple of times. She revealed that throughout my stay my physicians had been in contact with my parents. While my mother and father had never visited me, they had met with at least one of my physicians. My mother had indicated that she wanted nothing to do with me, that I had consistently lied to her and stolen from her. Moreover, she claimed that I had perennially done badly in school and that I had manufactured illnesses in the past to garner her attention. The social worker emphasized that it was important that I leave the hospital as soon as possible. My clinicians and parents concurred that it was time for "tough love," and that I would have to stop depending on my parents for support. I was to leave to spend three weeks with an old friend of the family, who apparently had also been separately warned not to offer me protracted assistance. Ostensibly, I did not need further medical follow-up or rehabilitation. This would only reinforce my attention-seeking behavior. What I needed was to get a job and to pull myself up by my proverbial bootstraps. Given what she said was my poor academic record, the social worker suggested that I seek some form of work, such as "becoming a bus driver." The message was very clear: I was to stop being a neurotic upper-class brat.

The social worker's tone battered me. I not only felt abandoned and betrayed but vilified. Her portrait of me was completely foreign. I stammered incoherently, not knowing where to begin to defend myself. I knew that I was a pretty good student. I offered to provide her with transcripts to prove my solid scholastic record. I reiterated my expectations of going on to professional or graduate school. She responded by saying that perhaps I should rethink my future as I obviously wasn't "strong" enough to undertake such endeavors. I think she was alluding to my lack of psychological and moral strength. I was completely taken aback and had no way to effectively respond.

When I left the hospital, my chart's diagnosis concluded rather ambiguously: "Right CVA. Conversion Reaction." CVA stands for cerebral vascular accident, or stroke. Right CVA locates the stroke as having happened in the right hemisphere of the brain. Conversion reaction was a replacement for the term "hysteria" in reference to psychosomatic disease during the 1980s. Other related terms in the mental health handbook of the time, the DSM-III,[1] that refer to psychosomatic illnesses

---

1. DSM-III stands for *Diagnostic and Statistical Manual of Mental Disorders*, third edition.

are: somatoform disorder, histrionic personality disorder, hypochondriasis, dissociative disorder, and disaffective disorder. All of these are considered to be personality disorders, which are considered to be some of the most chronic and intractable of mental illnesses. Individuals diagnosed with these syndromes are seen to be emotionally unstable, manipulative, narcissistic, and sexually or somatically obsessed.

But I had yet to fully comprehend the stigma and damage that the words "conversion reaction" would have in my medical chart.

6 Credo

After my discharge, I stayed for three weeks with a family I had known since I was four. And then I moved on. Fortunately, I had been able to arrange to rent a room in a house of friends near the university. Once there, I took over the master bedroom of the professor who was away on sabbatical. I unloaded a duffel bag of clothes into the bureau and tried to begin my life anew. My aim was to finish my undergraduate thesis, hold down some part-time jobs, and apply to graduate, law, and medical school for the following academic year. But underneath this veneer of plans, I remained shaken. Physically, I was frail. The muscles of my back and shoulders and hips were particularly weak, and by the end of the day, pain and fatigue seared through my body. One afternoon I was refused service at the corner grocer because my gait was so wobbly and my speech so slurred that the cashier assumed I was drunk. But my symptoms were uneven, quite literally, sometimes I had more movement and strength than at other times. This inconsistency disquieted me and made me wonder whether I was indeed delusional.

My friends, who were all in their early twenties, were kind but confused by my situation. Older family friends, many of whom I hadn't seen since I had left for boarding school as a young teenager, now called me and invited me to dinner. That first Christmas I was inundated with presents from these same people. One wealthy family lent me a computer for my remaining schoolwork; others wrote me good-sized checks, which helped me keep ahead of my bills. An American friend from boarding school paid my way to fly to New York for a week.[1]

In short, I became a cause célèbre. However, I felt shamed by my notoriety. I understood that people's good will arose out of sympathy for me, and I felt grateful for their efforts. But I wished that their interest in me arose out of a belief in the quality of my character and/or capacities, and I knew that most of them did not know me well enough for this to be true.

I felt shy. I spent most of my time working on my English undergraduate honors thesis. After much reading and pondering, an epiphany of sorts descended on me one evening as I sat in a pub. I sketched my thoughts on a paper napkin, graphically outlining an idea that became the backbone of my thesis. I met off and on with my supervisor. My work moved forward toward completion. One afternoon my supervisor informed me that a colleague had told him that nothing was really wrong with me and that I had faked my illness to get more time to finish my work. I felt hollow with disbelief as he recounted his story. In the end, with reddened cheeks, all I could do was deny it.

At different times I tried to return to athletics but discovered that my body simply gave out. I couldn't run or row or play squash. I did, on occasion, ride a bike. But when I crouched to lock it up, I usually discovered that I couldn't stand back up. Rest seemed to restore me. Nonetheless, my body remained capricious and unreliable. Late in the day I had more difficulties—my speech became slurred and I stumbled frequently. But despite my exhaustion and the strange poltergeist illness that lurked in me, I held a part-time job and finished my honors paper.

After a year, I received acceptances to graduate and law schools. Physically, it was clear to me that I could not meet the demands of first-year

---

1. U.S. Customs officers actually prevented me from getting on my plane because I was "disabled" and had too little cash with me. Rather ironically, they feared I might be seeking medical care in the United States that I could not pay for. My American friends vouched for me by phone, and I was allowed on the next flight. This was the first time I had ever been turned back at a border.

law school. I had seen friends logging huge hours in front of their legal textbooks. Even those with the best minds and work ethic seemed a little overwhelmed during midterms. I still found being up most of the day to be a grueling experience, often requiring me to stay in bed the following morning. I deferred my acceptances to law schools. In the meantime, I decided to enroll in a master's program in political science at the university from which I had just graduated. I suspected I could handle graduate classes; I assumed I could skip some as long as I kept up with reading and essay assignments. In my awareness that I neither had the stamina for full-time work nor for the rigors of professional school, a graduate degree seemed a safe and constructive option. At the same time, I also managed to get a bit more physical therapy at a new hospital. A lower-leg brace was made for my weaker side, which made walking easier—though it also made me self-conscious. I also switched psychiatrists and began to do intensive psychotherapy every day in an all-out effort to "recover" myself.

One afternoon, a philosophy professor invited me to accompany him on "grand rounds" at a local hospital. This session was to be entirely devoted to biomedical ethics. Although I have little memory of the topics discussed that morning, I do remember having a minor revelation of sorts. All of the lecturers were doctors. All of them had attended a six-week course on ethics at an American university, which apparently qualified them to throw about ambrosial terms such as "deontology" and "utilitarianism." As I sat and listened to these men—for the presenters were all men—they seemed to apply these philosophical ideas as though they were formulas that could be applied to different clinical situations. I had never heard philosophy discussed or treated in this manner. I had also been told in the car ride to the lecture that bioethics was an interdisciplinary field composed of an array of experts, such as doctors, nurses, philosophers, sociologists, and theologians. Apparently, they all contributed equally to this burgeoning new field. But it seemed to me that, given that only physicians spoke at this session, it was they who were making inroads into philosophy and not philosophers who were making inroads into medicine. In this way, then, doctors were not really being critiqued but were co-opting the very tools that might have been used by professionals outside the clinic to effectively criticize medical practices. Near the end of the rounds, I raised my hand to comment on what I had seen. My professor friend jumped on my arm and reminded me that I was only a guest—I was not empowered to speak. In the car, he smiled knowingly as I voiced my observations. It was at that moment I decided to write my master's thesis on issues of power in medicine.

When I began graduate school, I originally had asked permission to tape-record my classes. This was to save me the energy of trying to write notes and follow discussions. I did this for several weeks, but found that transcribing notes afterward from the tapes was too laborious. This strategy didn't really save my energy—in fact, it depleted my reserves. I realized that I was going to have to become a better listener—that I would need to rely less on written notes and more on a highly selective ear and on strengthening my memory.

My neurological symptoms still puzzled me. On my way to school, I passed a billboard for several weeks of which I could not decipher the relationship of the graphics to the text. It looked like a line drawing of an enormous upside down strawberry ice cream cone, and yet the words talked about feathers and dry cleaning. I would stop and puzzle over it daily when I went by. It was a few months before I finally figured out that the image was a logo of a pink flamingo, peeking out from behind plastic-wrapped shirts. I found instances of this type of spatial incoherence unsettling. Furthermore, I also retained my hypersensitivity to temperature and textures on certain parts of my body. (Ironically, my weak leg was almost always ice-cold to the touch.) For example, one day I tried to help a friend clear his parents' garden. I guided the rototiller a few feet, but the vibration proved too much and my hands and arms grew weak, numb, and began to swell. Despite the beautiful sunny morning, I had to sit down on an embankment to wait for normal movement and sensation in my limbs to return. All during this time, I desperately held on to an image of myself as young and fit, but a harsher reality kept running up against a self-aggrandized version of my former self. As a result, I often felt unreliable and incompetent because I was a very poor judge of my own physical capacities.

Oliver Sacks had just published *The Man Who Mistook His Wife for Hat,* and I found his neurological tales fascinating. By looking through the bibliography, I discovered the Soviet neurologist A. R. Luria's *The Man with a Shattered World* and *The Mind of a Mnemonist.* The first book is about the phantom pains of amputees. The second, however, intrigued me more. It recounts the life of a man with incredible memory but who lacks the capacity to synthesize meaning or emotion in his life. His hyperability is accompanied by corresponding deficits. This resonated with me. Moreover, Luria's descriptions of the mnemonist's tactics gripped me. The mnemonist creates an internal landscape and places each item or word in a list in it in such a way that it stands out—for example, he places a white egg against a red fire hydrant. All he has to do to recall something, even months later, is to walk through the mental panorama and pick out the variously placed pieces. If he does miss something, it is due to his having accidentally placed an egg against a white fence and thus he overlooks it when retracing his steps. All of this helped. I had found both my concentration and memory lagging—neuropsychological tests confirmed these weaknesses—but it wasn't clear to me whether these failures were due to psychological depression, lack of confidence, or neurological insult. But Luria's book taught me that I might bypass these weaknesses if I developed new strategies. I discovered that although my reading speed had slowed, my auditory memory had increased. I could remember ten-digit phone numbers after only dialing them once because they created both mathematical and auditory patterns for me. In an effort to stay abreast of my schoolwork, I took fewer and fewer notes and tried harder to organize and recall what I heard and read, arranging and rearranging the information in memorable matrices.

In spite of this, though, I found the workload more trying than I had before I was ill. Professors commented on my slurred speech when I was tired. Other graduate students formed reading groups, plowing through tertiary texts and authors together. But I couldn't keep up, and I dropped out of these gatherings. People went to bars and after-hours clubs together. I sometimes joined them but found myself slow and uncomfortable. I felt clumsy and was embarrassed by my fatigue and awkwardness.

Now, almost three years after my first incident of paralysis and in my early twenties, my inadequacies made me feel as though I had become less attractive. Previously, I had had such physical confidence that I felt no need to wear makeup because I believed my natural state was simply enough to be alluring. What may have seemed like an apathy toward feminine wiles was in fact a gross arrogance about my physical attractiveness. But, with fatigue, weak limbs, and a brace on the lower part of one leg, skirts seemed preposterous. My dress had always tended toward the tomboyish, and I now adopted wearing pants as a way of masking my deficiencies. I couldn't really dance at clubs anymore, and I worried that the recreational drugs that my peers experimented with might cause me further damage. I was unsure of myself and harbored a simultaneously fear of and longing for sexual contact. Contradictory signals emanated from me, which both pushed and pulled men and women from and toward me in social situations. On a couple of occasions I had one-night stands with young men who only vaguely appealed to me, one of which resulted in my getting a sexually transmitted disease. On other occasions, I dated an acquaintance from childhood who stood to inherit vast sums of money. I felt the censorious judgments of those who knew both of us that, given my newly disabled state and his social standing, I would not make him a suitable partner. I scuttled his interest by always inviting a friend to join us at the last minute. I also ended up in an affair with an older, married woman, who was incredibly kind and generous to me; but in the midst of it I fell deeply and unwisely in love with another young man. This passion was, in the end, largely unrequited. In sum, I was not a good or stable choice of romantic partner.

Despite my waverings, a group of young friends stuck by me; they shared meals and lodging with me, passed around notes from some of my classes, and put up with my litany of self-absorbed observations about my physical symptoms and complaints. On the periphery, a handful of older friends also endured the vagaries of both my physical state and my emotional inconstancy. It was the support of various combinations of these people that helped me navigate the next decade or so of ill health and disability.

My body ached and ached from being up during the day. In an effort to control the pain, I began to take over-the-counter acetaminophen with codeine. The dosage of two pills wasn't enough, and I often swallowed four or five at a time (sometimes more) to dampen the penetrating pain.[2] But I didn't tell my physicians or therapists about my discomfort because I thought that it would make me seem even more discreditable. For me the pain was illegitimate and thus not worthy of noting medically. As no one really understood why I was weak, complicating the picture by complaining about pain seemed ill-advised. When I visited the clinic, I focused on restoring my function. I didn't want to seem to whine.

By this time, I lived in a low-rent part of town at a considerable distance from the university. I tried to ride my racing bike (with my leg brace) for several weeks, but I found that my strength gradually wore away rather than built up. I used money from one of my student grants to buy a very small motorcycle—more of a glorified moped than a motorcycle—that gave me the freedom to move about the city and get to classes. My little scooter helped me ration my energy so that I could lead a more normal existence. I loved it and rode it through the snowy, slushy winter. It also had a "cool" factor, since it necessitated a black leather jacket, gloves, and a motorcycle helmet.

Academically, my new transportation and strategies paid off. I did well enough to gain admission to the Kennedy School of Government at Harvard and receive a number of fellowships. This coupled with my law school deferral and an interview for medical school gave me a number of choices. I decided that an Ivy League degree would give me the most professionally. But my scholarship would not be enough to support me. I made a misguided appeal to my grandparents and others for assistance but was rebuffed. I probed other scholarships and eventually secured another one as well as a bank loan. But as I made my preparations to move to Boston, I discovered that due to my ongoing medical care and my "preexistent

2. At the time I was unaware of the damage that chronic usage or high dosage of acetaminophen could do to my liver. I assumed that I could safely exceed what was probably a conservative dosage prescription on the box.

medical condition" I might not be covered by Harvard's health plan. I also fretted that my ongoing fatigue and my poltergeist of muscle weaknesses might hobble my studies. My mind was fit, but was the rest of me? I faced a dilemma. Should I risk moving to the United States without adequate health coverage? I might not experience any physical problems—perhaps my symptoms (if they were psychological) would resolve in the new environment. And even if they didn't, perhaps an American medical team (i.e., one from a private system) might take a fresh (and less condemning) approach to my ailments. I was unsure. Intuitively, I knew my illness was far more threatening and serious than the doctors who treated me made out. My body thus told me to be cautious. Would backing away from this opportunity mean that I was being too timid? Would it give my physical symptoms too much credence? Or was it wise to listen to what my body was telling me and choose a safer possibility?

Even as I turned down my admission, I felt like a coward. Instead, I took the fellowships I had and enrolled in a PhD program at my home university.

7 More Paralysis and More Psychological Remedies

In Toronto I continued the ongoing psychotherapy that I had engaged in for two years. Going five days a week had become emotionally addictive. The psychiatrist, Dr. D., espoused a view that if I totally committed myself to an in-depth relationship with him I would ultimately resolve all of my physical and psychological issues. He had taken on my case soon after I had restarted physical therapy at a new hospital. We connected well. The books on his bookshelves were many of the same on my own. Further, he encouraged me to explore any books that caught my eye and were new to me. He loved classical music as did I. He theorized that I had been insufficiently attached to my parents and thus needed to emotionally attach to him in order to gain psychological coherence. To a large extent, it worked. He and our sessions were never far from my thoughts as I pursued my scholarly life. On many occasions, he tried unsuccessfully to hypnotize me to rid me of my body's chronic paresis. But on we went: his asking, demanding, cajoling more stories of my past and myself, and my trying to recount every kernel I could remember and to recall every dream that washed up from my unconscious.

But the process worsened my depression. It dredged up unpleasant memories and bathed me over and over in the dramas and betrayals of my original family. The more work we did, the more I felt like a misfit in the land of the so-called psychologically normal. In fact, this constant chasing after elusive traumas (along with dealing with my physical symptoms) made me so depressed and unsure of myself that I almost became suicidal, and in one instance I was admitted to a psychiatric unit for a three-week stay.

When I got out, I continued my studies, which were going well. The department approved my master's thesis proposal, and my courses were also going well. I held down a part-time job at a local research institute. After I had worked there for a summer, my boss offered me a full-time position. Despite all my efforts, I worried that I was not physically ready for a forty-hour work week. I pondered the employment contract and then declined it. It killed me inwardly to be turning down opportunities that normally I would have been leaping at with enthusiasm. But my body continued to feel as though an unknown and dangerous menace stalked it. In short, despite the hours and hours of physical therapy and psychotherapy, my body remained weak, in pain, and unreliable.

I continued to surmise that pursuing a graduate degree remained the best vocational strategy.

Moreover, my worries about my physical robustness were made real, when, in the midst of my master's course year, I had an emergency appendectomy and awoke from the anesthetic, once again, with severe weakness and paralysis. Needless to say, when I found myself returned to an invalid state, my surprise was enormous. My vision was blurred, I had difficulty breathing, I couldn't sit up, and I was extremely exhausted.

As I recovered on the surgical ward, I could see the incredulity in the faces of the staff who cared for me. They knew that they had taken appropriate precautions to protect me from having another "stroke." Preoperatively, a cardiologist had examined me and declared me fit for surgery. The anesthesiologist had monitored my vitals with vigilance. And yet, I awoke in post-op with profound weakness. My psychiatrist visited the ward and demanded further medical investigations. Another MRI was ordered. But the scan proved to be negative. No one could understand what had happened: the lab results on my cerebrospinal fluid revealed atypical "oligloconal bands," which usually indicated some sort of neurologic abnormality (such as multiple sclerosis). In my case, these results—the same findings would be replicated a number of times over several years—were dismissed as uninterpretable because they were atypical in their presentation and thus "probably did not represent evidence of disease process."[1] Moreover, the diagnosis of psychosomatic illness (in the form of conversion reaction) now largely dominated my chart, and, for most medical staff, this opinion was reinforced by the fact that I saw a psychiatrist—which created a circularity to their reasoning: the patient may be psychosomatic, and so she should see a psychiatrist; and, since she sees a psychiatrist, she must be psychosomatic.

While my physicians remained largely congenial, they were obviously confounded. As the object of their bewilderment, I grew afraid. Not only was I utterly dismayed to be paralyzed again, but I also felt imminently threatened by the mysteriousness of my affliction. If no one knew what was wrong with me, no one could prevent it from happening again. I began to comprehend medicine's powerlessness in the face of uncertainty. Furthermore, I understood that if the cause of my illness remained unknown, my doctors would once again turn to my psyche as the root of my problem. However, I was no longer completely convinced that a purely psychological approach to my symptoms was going to restore my health. Throughout my tenure as a patient, I doubted that I was truly hysterical. As much as it seemed highly likely to my physicians, it seemed highly unlikely to me that I was ill simply to garner secondary gains and attention.

Nonetheless, the self-exploration of psychotherapy benefited me in many ways. It allowed me to give voice to the injuries of my familial past and to vent my frustration with my ongoing illness. However, it also exposed me to a myriad of assumptions and techniques that I found belittling. Psychotherapy as a form of medical treatment did not avoid the pitfalls of other clinical approaches. Despite its focus on personal narrative, its conclusions could be used to objectify me as a patient. It employed broad, generalizing theoretical frameworks for interpreting my life story. These theories seemed to me to be rather like pop psychology categories in lifestyle magazines; they were general enough that one could

---

1. This statement is from my medical chart at the time.

roughly interpret a life within its guidelines, but they were not specific enough to clearly reflect an individual's lived experience, understanding, and/or behavior. It appeared as though clinicians selectively chose which of their patient's life events were most important, highlighting the ones that fit a mental disease paradigm and glossing over those that did not. Ultimately, both of these aspects of psychotherapy diminished rather than increased my sense of personal agency. I began to view the psychologizing of my illness with increasing suspicion. It felt coercive.

For example, in my own case, the clinical significance of my relationship with my parents changed over time. Originally, my physicians regarded me as a wayward offspring of a reputable family. But within a year or two of psychotherapy, my mother and father became monstrous ogres. Rather than being someone who survived a lack of parental affection and concern, I was now seen as someone who was congenitally and fundamentally neurotic and unbalanced as a result of my parents' inability to form proper emotional attachments to me.

In an effort to escape from the clinical stereotyping of my past, and thus of my selfhood, I once lied when I was admitted to a hospital in which I had never been treated. I told the staff that my parents were dead. At the time, I thought it would be easier than attempting to justify their conspicuous absence. The concomitant shock, disapproval, and suspicion that arose every time I was asked to explain my parents' disinterest was profoundly frustrating. I had long ago acclimated myself to their antipathy, but continually having to satisfy others' (particularly clinicians') curiosity grew very tiring. This was especially true when I experienced very serious problems—I couldn't help but feel, as I lay in intensive care, that my physicians' attention should be less on my familial background and more on the immediate crisis at hand. Unfortunately, the medical staff at the new hospital discovered, through the faxing of my previous medical charts, that I had lied. (My stupidity in even thinking I could avoid my familial stigma was the result of poor judgment and extreme illness.) So now my doctors viewed me with even greater leeriness.

Even though I wasn't getting better, my psychiatrist insisted it was because we hadn't plumbed my emotional depths. A year passed. And another. And another. And another. As I discovered more and more about myself, I continued to have muscular paresis and serious relapses that landed me in the hospital repeatedly. I became a frequent flier at the local emergency room. Perhaps, my therapist suggested, I simply didn't trust the process enough. He tried hypnosis, which didn't work, and concluded that I was a poor hypnotic subject because my paralysis didn't disappear while I was in a trance. I argued in return that perhaps I *was* a good hypnotic subject and perhaps my paralysis was an indication that something was organically (and not functionally) wrong with me. Moreover, if he was correct in believing that I did not go into trance well, this was evidence that I did not possess one of the key features of psychosomatic patients (i.e., of being easily suggestible). Finally, I also argued that hypnosis wasn't considered to be a reliable therapeutic approach in the medical literature. He dismissed my critiques as being "too intellectual" and that a major part of my problem was that I was "too intelligent." (Doctors would accuse me of this a number of times over the next decade, intimating that I might be confounding them with my symptoms as some sort of intellectual game.) Ironically, the predominant psychiatric treatment manual (i.e., the DSM) states that psychosomatic patients are often uneducated and come from less cosmopolitan environments. My discussions with Dr. D. thus frustrated and confused me. And my psychogenic diagnosis seemed to be a maze from which I could not extricate myself.

When I began to read up on the creation and maintenance of psychiatric diagnoses, I discovered that until the 1980s one of the pervading difficulties in psychiatry was that practitioners only agreed about diagnoses 20 percent of the time. Despite employing a discourse of objectivity, psychiatric diagnoses thus had no statistical or scientific reliability. A young psychiatrist at the time, Robert Spitzer, decided that the diagnostic manual was at fault and set about to revise it. He created more than two dozen committees to write detailed descriptions of psychiatric disorders. Because there was little research at the time, the committees arrived at definitions through often chaotic debate. Spitzer would take notes at these meetings and then set about summarizing various disorders. He alone decided which opinion weighed more heavily in any definition. As such, the *Diagnostic and Statistical Manual of Mental Disorders,* third edition (DSM-III), published under his leadership, did not have diagnoses that were scientifically derived. However, the new manual was far more comprehensive than previous ones and provided a means for psychiatrists to be more consistent in their application of terms, thereby producing more reliability in the field of mental health diagnoses.

Given the idiosyncratic manner in which the DSM is composed, it is not surprising that the descriptions are often vague and opaque. The DSM has been revised twice since Spitzer's first efforts. And its chair is now an esteemed position within psychiatry. Nonetheless, from a strictly scientific point of view, the composition of diagnoses is still highly politicized. Paula Caplan, the psychologist who sat on some of the American Psychiatric Association's committees when the DSM-III-R and DSM—IV were being prepared, argues that the DSM lacks the scientific authority to which it lays claim (Caplan 1995). She uses two examples, "self-defeating personality disorder" and "pre-menstrual dysphoric disorder," to demonstrate the haphazard manner in which diagnoses are delineated. Her main argument is that psychiatric diagnostic categories are largely the result of amorphous and politicized discussions. Their scientific bases reside only in the effort to create "reliable" categories for practitioners to agree on, and the content of these categories is, for the most part, untested by methodologically valid research. Caplan adroitly argues that even those studies that point to the DSM's efficacy in improving reliability in diagnosis are skewed by the presence of highly obvious diagnoses such as substance abuse disorders; less conspicuous (and far more numerous) labels have only about 50 percent reliability between differing diagnosticians, a low rate for statistical validity.

More generally in medicine a distinction exists between illnesses that are thought to be "organic" (i.e., originating in the body) and "functional" (i.e., originating in the psyche). Physicians thus categorize patients according to whether they can find physical evidence of disease. Medical journals report that up to a third of patients present with psychosomatic symptoms—and that this is particularly true in neurological practices. So, when an individual is sick without apparent medical cause, the practitioner refers the individual to a counselor or psychiatrist in order to deal with stress-induced or functional symptoms. In the past, such illnesses were known as "hysteria" or "Briquet's syndrome." Today, hysteria, per se, as a diagnostic category no longer exists. The DSM-IV speaks instead of "hysterical personality disorder," "somatization disorder," "conversion disorder," "dissociative disorder," and/or "anxiety hysteria" in categorizing such ailments. (Malingering is thought to be a distinct and separate entity since it is a conscious fabrication of symptoms.) All of these labels try to capture those patients who exhibit "abnormal illness behavior" and whose complaints do not seem to bear out under investigation. But cultural stereotypes persist despite the new summaries, often contradicting themselves—coquettish women, Mediterranean and/or effete men, and sexually repressed females are all considered likely candidates for psychogenic illnesses. And so, even though hysteria has disappeared from the official parlance of the clinic, conceptually it has never gone away—it remains in the characterization of somatoform and dissociative disorders.

New diagnostic terminologies do not obviate the presence of sexual metaphor in the clinical assessment of psychosomatic illness. There is good evidence that physicians perceive women's maladies to be largely the result of emotionality, and thus they give little credence to women's suffering (Smith 1992, 31–32). If doctors understand little about women and/or believe that their ailments are psychosomatic, then it seems likely that they will ignore women's complaints or treat them as aberrant. A persistent cultural association of emotional lability with women means that they're diagnosed with somatoform disorders more often than men.

While physicians know that men, particularly combat soldiers, suffer from psychosomatic diseases, they tend to employ terms such as "neurasthenia," "shell shock," "combat fatigue," and "nervous exhaustion" to describe their symptoms. American and British veterans of the Persian Gulf War of the early 1990s suffer from a multiplicity of problems ranging from impotence and fatigue to respiratory and motor problems. They have "Gulf War syndrome." Thus far, no organic basis for the soldiers' symptoms exists. U.S. and British governments perceive the syndrome as a manifestation of psychological stress from fighting in a potential chemical-war battle zone. Alternatively, doctors believe that civilian men who suffer from somatoform disorders tend to be young, effeminate, immigrants, or poorly educated. The DSM-IV states: "Somatization Disorder occurs only rarely in men in the United States, but the higher reported frequency in Greek and Puerto Rican men suggests that cultural factors may influence the sex ratio." (DSM-IV, 447). This characterization reveals the ethnic bias of the manual and the North American propensity to stereotype "Mediterranean" men as more emotionally labile—that is, more feminine—than their male counterparts elsewhere. With regard to "conversion disorder," the manual reports that it is found more commonly in rural populations and developing regions (DSM-IV, 455). But the paradigm that people with psychosomatic disorder lack sophistication is not always true. Current literature also reports that nurses, medical students, and those with disabled family members are potential candidates for somatoform disorders. This is because they have a specialized knowledge of certain diseases that they can then unconsciously mimic with great accuracy. But it is very important to note that the unstated implication is that even the apparently "sophisticated" person with a psychosomatic disorder has obviously rudimentary psychological defenses, otherwise he or she would not fall prey to such a disorder.

To some extent psychological theories of disease are very attractive in liberal societies such as ours, because they posit the idea that individuals have mental and psychological control over their bodies. This means that we can truly be autonomous beings—we do not have to succumb to illness if we don't want to. Good health becomes a matter of willing oneself to be well. All sorts of apocryphal stories exist in our culture about people facing dire illnesses who laugh themselves or pray themselves or work themselves into such a state that they defeat their diseases. These tales fit beautifully with the liberal paradigm of free, autonomous people who can construct their own lives without limitation. Within this paradigm, we are not limited by our bodies or by our mortality. But this is a falsehood because, of course, we are mortal—we will die and we will inevitably become ill.

I had liked Ayn Rand's novels as a young adolescent, and so the idea that I should be able to heal myself was very appealing. A good, strong, and emotionally whole person—read, an ideal, liberal individual—should be able to overcome his or her physical (and psychological) ailments. Moreover, as my illness continued to progress, doctors began to hint that they needed to consciously "gatekeep" my access to health care resources, since my sickness was not real and health care was provided at public expense. Since I was a political scientist, these implications unfortunately affected me, and I sometimes wondered whether I was being a bad citizen because I wasn't getting well. At other times, though, I wondered whether I was actually receiving my due within the nationally and provincially funded health-care system. I thought that many doctors were denigrating my social membership and political equality when they chose to dismiss or belittle my symptoms. (I sometimes speculated that perhaps I might receive better care in the private health-care system in the United States. Any illusions I had about this were eventually dissolved when I received comparable treatment in American facilities later on in the course of my illness.) Psychologizing my illness thus damaged my self-esteem at a number of levels and at a time when I needed increased emotional strength to cope with my physical deterioration.

In addition, during the first five to seven years of my illness, Dr. D., my psychiatrist, encouraged me to yield myself to his care, often claiming that he was a superior substitute for my family of origin and that it was natural for me to "love" him. But, as I became sicker, I found that he was a poor substitute for the emotional sustenance of an *actual* family. The resurgence of my paralysis after my appendectomy (and the ensuing prolonged hospitalization and rehab) meant that I understood that he was not kin. His commitment to me was a professional one, and despite our seeming "friendliness," we were not even friends. It was a mistake to believe the rhetoric that remaining emotionally attached and devoted to our sessions would somehow provide me with the emotional sustenance I needed to navigate my illness and ultimately defeat it. I began to realize that I needed to either fall in love with or love someone who could properly reciprocate my feelings and actually thereby become my kin. At least then I would have a properly balanced relationship from which I could draw psychological and spiritual strength even as my body failed me.

8 A Pyrrhic Victory

But I've gotten ahead of myself. Let me go back to when I was twenty-two years old and I lay on a surgical recovery ward with profound paresis for a second time (after my appendectomy). I not only suffered from the physical discomfort of my incapacity but also felt utterly alone. I grasped that my caregivers viewed my presence with suspicion and disfavor. The young surgeons who had operated on me had to present my case at "M & M" (morbidity and mortality) rounds in which their actions were reviewed by superiors and peers in the hospital. Despite their affable banter, neither was pleased to be exposed to this type of scrutiny—especially given the underlying suspicion that my weakness was a fabrication of my psyche.

From my perspective, I was a prisoner, once again, in a hospital bed. But this time I understood what lay ahead and I wanted to jump-start my recovery. I struggled with my stronger arm to pull my body around on top of the bed. While still on the surgical recovery ward I asked for a bar to be suspended above my head. Within a day, a triangle of metal suspended on a metal chain arrived at my bedside. With some badgering I coaxed an orderly into hanging it. With my stronger arm I could grab it and use it to shift my weight a centimeter or so across the plastic-covered mattress. This meant that I was slightly less dependent on the nursing staff to move me, and I hoped that being able to shift myself, even slightly, might protect me from bedsores. I also worried that my feet were developing "foot drop." (Foot drop occurs when the weight of blankets and sheets force a weak or paralyzed foot into a semi–toe point position.) If left alone, my Achilles tendon would become too shortened and tight for me to walk properly once my strength returned.

Of course, I vainly hoped that my strength would return quite suddenly and I would be able to leap out of bed. I kept praying that every morning my muscles would wake up and respond to my commands. Each day, I demanded that the nurses dress me in my street clothes: a proper shirt (even if unironed), khakis or jeans, socks and shoes. I didn't want to feel or look like a patient. Internally, I refused to see myself as "sick"; rather, I took a mechanistic approach to my weakness and viewed it as something malfunctioning in me physically—if only I could unearth what it was!

But mostly I wanted to cry out at being trapped yet again by the weight and inertia of my body. Nonetheless, I pushed back my tears with an impatient anger. All I wanted to do was to stand up and flee. I felt that the incision in my abdomen was fairly innocuous compared to the paresis in my torso and limbs. The wound healed well, and I ignored the pulling of the staples as I tried over and over to lift myself into a sitting position or to roll myself in bed. Despite my efforts, the nurses needed to continue to lift, turn, and reposition me. Also, I was totally dependent on them for toileting, which I found belittling.

The weeks drained away, and the summer moved into late August. Eating remained exhausting, and a constant nausea plagued me most days. Even as I contemplated the ripening of my favorite fruit—peaches—I couldn't eat them. Friends brought me fruit baskets, and they sat on the windowsill simultaneously luring and sickening me.

One weekday afternoon, I was transferred to the rehabilitation unit. I took this as a positive sign. I would now receive the intensive physical and occupational therapy I needed to get me home. The next morning, my new occupational therapist came to see me. I knew of her already from when I had attended outpatient therapy the previous year. She was an outspoken Asian woman who tended to get into loud arguments with the rather irascible physician in charge of the unit. When I heard her coming down the hall, I worried that she would turn in at my doorway.

Her first words to me were: "What the hell are you doing here!" And then she quickly covered her mouth with the palm of her hand, "I...I...I mean 'heck.' I mean I didn't expect to see you! I don't know your name." She looked stunned, "Weren't you working with Donna a few months ago?"

I nodded.

"Weren't you walking?" She slipped down onto the arm of the chair beside my bed.

I nodded again, tears filling my eyes.

"So what are you doing here?"

I didn't know what to say. I was paralyzed. I couldn't even sit up, let alone walk. Swallowing and speaking were even difficult. But according to the MRI and the CT scan and all my blood work, there was nothing wrong with me. In the muddle and confusion of these intersecting thoughts I simply said, "I'm paralyzed again." One or two tears slipped underneath my eyelids and dribbled down my cheeks.

She leaned forward, "Don't worry. It's okay." She patted my arm. "You know who I am, right? I'm Jane." She stood up and took down the bed rail. "Can you scoot over?"

I reached up for the monkey bar and tried to slide myself across the sheets. I shifted one or two centimeters.

She leaned over me and grabbed me by my hips, "Okay, on three, we'll try it again. One...two...three."

And over I slid.

"There. Now, see if you can straighten yourself from the waist up."

I rocked back and forth from side to side, trying to align my torso and legs.

"Okay, let me help you. Grab my shoulder with your stronger hand. That's right. Now, pull on me as I reposition you. Good. There." Jane sat down on the edge of the bed facing me. "Now, what do you think I can help you with?"

"Well, I know you can help me with dressing and things. But what I really want is to be able to go to the bathroom by myself."

"Hmmm."

"No, really." I pleaded, "I really, really want to go to the bathroom by myself. It's bad enough being like this." I grabbed at my trouser leg with contempt. "But having someone else take me to the bathroom. I *hate* it!"

"I see what you mean. Well, there's only one accessible bathroom on the floor and it's down the hall."

"I'll go there. I don't care. As long as I can go by myself."

"Well, let me go find a wheelchair and I'll see what we can do." Within a few minutes Jane returned with a wheelchair. "We'll have to set you up with a proper one tomorrow—one that fits you better and has an air-cell cushion." She unclipped the arm off one side and slipped it in beside the bed. "Here is a transfer board. See if you can slide down on it."

With her help and a bit of gravity I eventually ended up in the chair. We replaced the armrest, and I wheeled myself slowly down the corridor. Once inside the bathroom, Jane stood back: "Now let's see what you can do."

I fiddled with the clip at the base of the armrest, trying to ease the tube out of its resting place. After a few minutes, I managed to free it, and the arm fell to the tile floor with a clatter. I reddened at the loud noise.

"Don't worry about that," she assured me. "Keep going."

I put my better arm on the seat of the toilet and tried to lift myself across the breach. I remained stationary: "Shit." I tried again. And again. And again. I grabbed at the handrail on the wall and, holding fast, attempted to pull myself onto the toilet. I felt my hips lift slightly. I pulled again. Again, a little bit more movement. My head and back and chest stung with fresh perspiration. I let my torso flop down onto my lap and, then pushed my head down to my knees so that my pelvis would rise (a trick I had learned from my first bout of paralysis). I pulled one last hard tug on the grab bar.

Jane stood in front of me. "Whoa! Whoa, whoa!" She braced her hands and legs so that they caught me as I careened toward the floor: "Not like that." Grabbing my pants on either side of my waist, she heaved me back into the chair. She crouched down beside my slumped figure, "So...have you had enough?"

I shook my head. I reached again for the handrail. I tried over and over and over. I fell into Jane's grasp at least three more times. On my final attempt, my vision had become blurred and my shirt, saturated. But on the final attempt, I managed to just slip onto the lip of the toilet. Gasping for breath, I hauled myself centimeter by centimeter until I was centered on the seat. From underneath my hunched torso and through my breathlessness, I hissed triumphantly, "See!"

Jane, still crouching beside me protectively, said, "Yeah, I see." She paused, her voice betraying a slight smile, "But tell me—how are you going to get your pants down?"

I swore streams of obscenities internally, but could only muster a weak, "Fuck!" I shook my bowed head. "Okay," I conceded.

"Here, let me help you." Jane reached around my back in an awkward hug. "On three back to the chair. One…two…three."

And I was back in the chair. Hunched over, I stared at the tile floor in defeat. Jane had read me correctly and had allowed me to find my limits—and how profoundly I felt them. No matter what the physicians believed, I could not just override this paralysis with will, nor with jovial good nature. With or without a diagnosis, I and I alone had to face its torment.

She wheeled me to my room, "Let's get you back to bed. You look exhausted." At my bed, she reached for the call bell, "Can someone come down to help me get this patient back to bed?" As we waited, she turned to me and said, "Tomorrow, I'll take you to the gym. We'll do an assessment and then get to work. And when you're ready, I promise we'll work on the toilet routine."

When they lifted me back into bed, my body sagged heavily into the mattress. I couldn't lift my head from the pillow. My damp shirt was stripped away and replaced with a hospital gown.

"Which way do you want to lie: facing the door or facing the window?"

"Window."

They rolled me over and lifted me onto my side. Jane placed a pillow between my legs and another at my back to prevent me from flopping backward. She beckoned the nurse, "Put this pillow under her arm there, her shoulder looks as though its subluxating." She tucked a final one behind my shoulder blades and neck. She pinned the call bell to the blanket, "There, the call bell is right beside your thumb."

The next day an orderly appeared. He lifted me ably into a wheelchair and pushed it into the hallway. He parked it with its brakes on so that I faced a wall spattered with hospital grime. I resented his oversight and tried to undo the brake lever but my hand was too weak. Downstairs, I was parked yet again, this time in a row of other patients who were all waiting for therapists to retrieve them. We sat lined up along one wall along a lengthy hallway facing the elevators. People rushed by us as though we were furniture. Occasionally, a therapist would shout out to someone in line as they wheeled another patient away, "Hey there, Mr. G!" But she or he would usually be gone before a reply was uttered.

When Jane came out to get me, she undid my brakes and let me wheel slowly into the gym. The room was about half the size of a basketball court and lit by fluorescent bulbs. Raised plinths with thick plastic mats ringed its outer edge. About ten patients, all older than me, were lying, sitting, or standing in various poses around the room. I was by far the youngest. We stopped in front of a plinth in the nearest corner. Jane unclipped my armrest and placed a wooden transfer board as a bridge between my right hip and the plinth. "Now let's try to get you over onto the mat. I'm going to help you a bit so you have some strength for the rest of the session."

Confronted by the indignity of exposing my awkwardness and inability to the patients around me, I couldn't speak or move. Tears filled my eyes. All I wanted to do was escape.

Jane quickly sat down opposite me, "What? What? You think these people care about what you do?" She put a hand on my knee. "They're too busy with their own stuff to worry about you. So stop being embarrassed. No one's interested in what you're doing." She paused, her eyes searching my face. "You take a second and then let's get on with it."

After a moment, I blocked out my self-consciousness and we transferred onto the mat. For the next forty minutes or so, Jane flexed, pushed, pulled, stretched, and notated my strengths and deficiencies. Rehab was simultaneously a place of hope and of potential disappointment. I wanted to get better, but would I? Plus I still didn't know what was wrong with me.

I approached physical and occupational therapy as though they were a form of athletic training. But speech therapy stymied me. Coordinating my tongue and jaw and swallowing were difficult. My words became slurred quite easily, especially as the day wore on. But I found it debasing to sit reciting sounds such as "Aka, ka, ka" or "pitika, pitika, pitika." I found my speech deficits to be particularly humiliating. Having a mirror thrust in front of me made the whole experience even more trying. Fortunately, as the weeks passed, my vocal control improved. As my body began to stir and I relearned specific movements, some of my joints began to swell. My efforts to stand and walk were complicated by pain in my knees and ankles. X-rays revealed that I had indications of arthritis in one or two of my joints. The blood work for rheumatoid arthritis did not reveal sufficient levels of antibodies, but the physical evidence indicated that an autoimmune disorder might lie at the root of my problems. Consequently, I underwent tests for lupus. But again, I didn't meet the diagnostic criteria.

As my stamina gradually improved, I also tried to keep up with my schoolwork. Even though my scholastic achievements brought me great solace, my doctors viewed them with suspicion. The physiatrist (rehab specialist), Dr. E., who ran the ward, questioned me one day about why it was taking me so long to get a PhD. He reprimanded me for falling behind my peers and for not completing my research within a year. I argued with him. My fieldwork was a little delayed because of my hospitalization, but all the rest of my work was on schedule. I would probably only need an extra term to finish my master's before going on to my doctoral program. Dismissing me with an impatient wave of his hand, he compared me to the young physicians who worked under his tutelage who would earn their medical "subspecialty" within a year or two and come away with a PhD behind their names. But the world of social sciences research was wholly different from that of the hospital. Furthermore, the Canadian academic system treated the MA as a distinct degree from either the BA or PhD. The route to doctoral candidacy was thus much longer and more involved than he imagined. But nothing I said could convince him that I wasn't a professional laggard.

My physical progress was steady but slow. Although symptoms worsened with fatigue as the day progressed, I was slowly climbing my way back into a stronger state. After many weeks, I started to stand and walk. My gait, however, was still erratic. I could walk short distances at a moderate to slow speed but couldn't increase my pace without having my torso muscles give out and buckle me forward. My physiotherapist encouraged me to walk to a metronome as she gradually increased the cadence. Nonetheless, my proximal weakness hindered any improvements. But my arms and hands improved and so did my speech, even if it was slurred when I was tired. The staff and I began to plan for my discharge.

Jane, the occupational therapist, left the clinic a few weeks before then to work elsewhere. My new occupational therapist (OT) would be responsible for ensuring that I went home with appropriate skills and equipment. I could now bathe, dress, and toilet myself. She assessed my cooking skills. We also decided that I would need a wheelchair for long distances—something that I knew to be reasonable but that utterly depressed me. My weakness still affected my left side more profoundly than my right. I couldn't fully raise my left arm. My left leg, back, and stomach muscles were weaker than those on my right side. Consequently, the OT prescribed a "hemi-height" folding wheelchair that was usually prescribed for stroke patients. I found it uncomfortable and heavy. My back and shoulder ached terribly after using it only a short time. Years of athletic training on bicycles had taught me that rigid, light frames transferred one's expended energy more directly to the wheels and to the movement of the bicycle. I applied this same principle to the wheelchair and asked for a lighter, more rigid chair. My request was rebuffed. Apparently, such innovations were "sports chairs" and only for those with spinal cord injuries. The staff implied that I was adopting a crippled role that was inappropriate. The belief was that only true cripples (i.e., those who could not walk for valid reasons) had the right to high-end equipment. I did not belong to this group.

Once home, I discovered that the wheelchair they had prescribed was too heavy for me to lift up the four steps of the front porch and down the narrow passageway into the house. A friend welded a small metal shed at the curbside that could store the folded frame. Despite this improvement, when I went to the shops three blocks away, my arm, shoulder, and back ached so badly that I held back tears on the way home. After two to three months of enduring this pain, I felt trapped at home. I had no car. My muscles could no longer manage my small motorcycle. The wheelchair exhausted and pained me so that going out became a real trial.

I bitched and bitched about the wheelchair, which increasingly sat in its little metal hutch out in the snow. A fellow graduate student very generously lent me a car for two to three days a week. This allowed me to go to the library and attend lectures. On a cold February day, I approached a young woman who was sitting in a sports wheelchair outside the library waiting for a ride. Tentatively, I asked her about her rigid-frame chair. She gave me the name and phone number of the vendor. The following day I called him and arranged to meet him at his office in the east end of the city. Within an hour he had set me up with a "demo" chair to try. The wheels quick-released off the sides, and the back folded down onto the seat. As I lifted it into the backseat of the car, I wondered rapturously about its feather-weight design.

The chair transformed my life. In the end, an old family friend gave me the money to purchase it—an offer I simply couldn't refuse. I could lift the chair relatively easily into the house I shared with another student, a writer, and an artist. More important, I could wheel it with relative comfort moderate distances and even up a slight incline. I gained liberty with its use. I could now go out with friends, go to the store, and spend longer hours at the university. Some evenings, I even went to dance at after-hours clubs with my housemates. I still felt awkwardly conspicuous sitting in a wheelchair, however, and I reddened at meeting new people or at well-meaning offers of assistance. I withdrew socially even as I desperately wanted to be carefree and popular. Fatigue and pain were a constant presence. On my evenings to make dinner, I often ended up crouching beside the stove to prepare the meal because I found static standing to be so tiring that I sometimes felt faint. I bowed out of collective chores and social outings.

To others, I appeared narcissistic and self-preoccupied—which I was. Unfortunately, I felt unable to confide wholly in anyone, and thus my partial confidences to friends were confusing and inconsistent. I relied on friends and housemates enormously. By sheer proximity, they stood in for my family—a burden that they neither wanted nor deserved. I knew that I was wearing out relationships, but I couldn't do anything to stop it. Internally, my sense of self ranged chaotically from false bravado to vanquished victim. The disintegration of my own life preoccupied me in a way that made me all but incapable of tending to others' needs. As friends withdrew, either silently or by more overt declarations, my sense of feeling wounded and abandoned grew.

I felt barely in control. When I had both the mental and physical energy, I probed the university's medical library, asking for articles to be pulled on everything from neurological paralysis to hysterical conversion. I read the anatomy and physiology texts of one of my lovers. In short, I tried to puzzle out what might be at the root of my ongoing debility and pain, but failed.

My romantic relationships foundered. As one ended, I would lurch into another ill-conceived liaison in which I doubted my sexual attractiveness and as a result doubted the partner who was attracted to me. The typical amorous insecurities of youth were amplified and conflated by my own confusion about my body and psyche. Throughout these years, I pushed and pulled lovers in and away—never quite believing that I was attractive and unconsciously putting down those who seemed to be drawn to me anyway.

Academically, my doctoral program went well. I won a prestigious fellowship that guaranteed multiyear funding. My topic focused on "applying moral and philosophical theory to real-life situations" (increasingly I thought I would focus on medicine); it intrigued me, and I relished hours spent reading, probing, and thinking. I put an extension cord on my computer keyboard and perched my monitor at the end of my bed so that I could work lying down. I also finally bought a small television so that I resented less the many hours that I spent lying in my room.

9 *Becoming a Pariah*

I was now twenty-four, and my life had resumed a rhythm of sorts, until one morning when I bent over to tie my shoes and my stomach suddenly rushed down my throat and emptied onto the carpet. I hadn't actually vomited. It was as if a portal had suddenly opened up and my body just let go of the food it was digesting. I thought little of it, until it happened again a few days later. During this period I fell ill with yet another bout of pneumonia. I took a course of antibiotics but then had another round a couple of weeks later. My general practitioner suspected that the upper sphincter of my stomach was allowing fluid to slide up my throat and into my lungs. Tests seemed to support this theory. Over the next few months, however, eating and swallowing became more difficult. I had more incidents of bizarre stomach emptying. I steadily lost weight.

Psychologically, I was ambivalent about continuing the almost daily psychotherapy with Dr. D. I felt we had reached an impasse. Clearly, the work wasn't paying off. I was no better.

As the summer ebbed, I grew thinner. My general practitioner arranged for me to have a variety of gastroenterological tests. This, along with dehydration, required me to make two short hospital stays. The tests revealed little. During one of them, I had a nasty reaction to a small dose of Haldol—normally a psychiatric drug for psychosis—which had been administered to me to prevent my ongoing nausea. It gave me a horrible sense of muscular irritability in which all I wanted to do was keep moving, while my weakness prevented me from pacing back and forth. The internal tension in my whole body was almost unbearable. After a few hours, its effects thankfully wore off. But despite my protestations, I was given another intravenous dose during the night, making my next hours sheer misery. The staff seemed largely unsympathetic. Confronted by their apparent indifference and even mild hostility, part of me hoped that whatever was wrong with me would kill me off quickly or that I would simply get better.

A friend, who was a young physician, invited me to her family home for a seaside holiday and, despite my usually anxieties, I decided to go. Her parents and many siblings embraced me warmly. Their house hummed with energy. Her father, who was a doctor, suggested that I go to the local hospital for a few tests to discover the source of my weight loss. The prospect of a fresh medical start in which my symptoms would not be presumed to be psychogenic tempted me, and, after some persuasion, I agreed.

I was admitted to the hospital, and a scoping of my stomach revealed that the sphincter was in fact a little lax. But more important, it revealed that my stomach was static. My digestive system was processing food so slowly that I was becoming malnourished. But the cause of these problems remained elusive. The staff performed a variety of tests—including ones for the autoimmune disease scleroderma. Everything came back negative, which was as paradoxical as it was frustrating—most people would be happy to discover that "there's nothing wrong with you."

On the one hand, I wanted to be well regardless of the diagnosis. On the other, I wanted to have a specific disease—an entity that could be identified, named, and treated. If I had no diagnosis then my symptoms meant nothing—which in this case reinforced the view that I was a nut case, full stop. Since something was really wrong, the two impulses contradicted each other. Intellectually, I decided that I should just focus on getting well and ignore the issue of causation. But emotionally I wanted to be validated—I wanted my illness to be judged real. I wanted my symptoms to be visible so that a clinician could finally and accurately diagnose their meaning.

As I look back on this episode, I believe that my emotional needs prolonged my malaise both unconsciously and consciously. It is true that even now when I go into a "neurological crisis" my digestive system often shuts down, making even tube feedings difficult or impossible to sustain me, but I am also aware that this period of prolonged digestive stasis was one in which my psychological self was also vibrating in a state of indecision and unknowing—my psychological self was in symbiosis with my physical state.

Because I was not digesting food well, my muscles grew even weaker. I found it increasingly difficult to move or to walk. Having ascertained that my stomach absorbed few nutrients, the gastroenterologist decided to start me on intravenous feeding—or parenteral nutrition. I was fitted with a central line—a large type IV tube that attaches through the chest wall to a large vein. A complicated schedule of hanging bags of sugar, proteins, minerals, and lipids ensued. Within a day or two I felt much, much better. I could almost sense the uptake of nutrition into my tissues.

At the same time, the doctors decided that they wanted to move me back to Toronto to finish up my recovery. They quickly discovered that few hospitals, if any, were interested in accepting a transfer. My friend's father came in one morning seething with frustration, "Don't worry. I won't give up. We will find a way to get you home." He walked back and forth in front of me for a few more seconds. "There is one more thing I should tell you. I would stay away from that psychiatrist, Dr. D. He said terrible things about you. Really terrible things. I'd stay away from him; he is no friend of yours!"

His words hit me. I felt my cheeks and chest redden with hurt and shame. Dr. D. and I had disagreed many times. Of late, I had certainly struggled in the psychotherapy process, but I had not conceived that he thought badly of me—or that he would speak ill of me—I presumed we held each other in mutual respect. I had misjudged and misread both him and our relationship. I felt stupid and humiliated by the fallibility of my trust.

Once again, I had become a medical annoyance. When clinicians came to see me their frustration was palpable. In my indecision, I was unsure whether I wanted to go back to a hospital in Toronto—my medical chart so deeply sullied my reputation in those clinics. In a moment that I still deeply regret and that still brings a flush of shame to my face when I recall it, I deliberately infected the IV site on my chest. I vomited one morning and did not clean away a portion of it that slipped into the partially open side of the bandage covering the wound. Even as I chose to let this happen, I knew it was stupid and wrong; but I did it anyway. I believed that I might forestall my transfer, in the vain hope that a clearer clinical picture might emerge. Despite the plethora of diagnostic testing that revealed little about the cause of my weakness, I instinctively knew that something was wrong with me. Moreover, I still believed that medicine could uncover it and provide some sort of validity for my appalling physical state. Paradoxically, the induced infection was an act of faith—faith in my physicians' capacity, if given more time and more investigation, to discover what was wrong with me.[1] It was a psychological torment to be suffering so much physical pain and debility without any legitimate cause. I'd worked terribly hard in the rest of my life to behave honorably, and I did not want to continue to be seen as a medical outlaw. Unfortunately, the infection likely did the opposite: once the site was swabbed, my subterfuge was probably revealed. No one said anything to me. But a certain silence descended around my care from which I grasped that I had become a clinical felon. My transfer was quickly affected—to (unknown to me) a chronic care ward for Alzheimer's patients in Toronto. Understandably, I never heard from my young doctor friend or her family again.

I was returned to a Toronto hospital whose buildings were a chaotic mixture of old and new structures, organized down a central spine of corridor that seemed to extend over a mile in length. I silently dubbed it the

---

1. I had little understanding at the time of how infections worked or were detected. It seems laughable now that I thought growing yet another culture from my cells might show something new. In retrospect, I'm sure that I was tested for all sorts of possible infections in the years previously. But I was desperate and emotionally at sea. Even if I had understood, I'm not sure my reason would have prevailed over my impulsive self.

"battleship clinic." But even as I tried to be internally witty, the hospital stay was awful. The wing to which I was admitted was physically rundown and overflowing with very elderly patients. The hallways and rooms were dimly lit and smelly.

Clinically, I was largely ignored. My first placement was in a four-bed ward that was so small that the beds were shoved together in pairs in the center of the room. I could quite literally reach out and touch the person in bed next to me. Not that I wanted to as my roommates were elderly demented women. The bathroom was down the hall and was shared by several rooms on the floor. The scent of stale urine and disinfectant dominated the unit. On arriving, I asked for a physiotherapy consult to make me stronger and to plan my discharge. But, instead, the IV feedings were withdrawn, and, as I grew weaker, I was told that rehab was unavailable.

Fortuitously, during the same month a publicly subsidized wheelchair apartment in downtown Toronto was offered to me. My name had been put down on the waiting list during one of my early bouts of paralysis three years earlier. Feeling miserable and confronted by my failing health, I signed the lease. Three friends set about packing up my room in the house I shared midtown. They then moved my belongings to my new apartment downtown in the financial district. I felt intuitively that my housemates of many years were relieved to see me, and my things, depart. They had endured more than enough of physical illnesses, crises, narcissism, and disability. But more important, for the first time, it would be possible for me to go home, even if I wasn't walking well (or at all!).

After lingering in the ward room for a couple of weeks, I managed to contact the hospital's admitting department and get moved to a private room on the floor, as I had private health coverage. This infuriated my attending physician, Dr. H. She seldom came to see me. But when she did she adopted a contemptuous and aloof manner. The most contact we had was when she chastised me one day for maintaining relationships with "people of stature" in the community. Dr. H. glowered at me, "Don't you understand you're an inappropriate drain on these people?" She named a couple of friends of my parents' generation who continued to visit me. One of them sat on the hospital's board. "You are not their family member! You do understand that don't you?!" She paused, her left hand on her hip, defiantly, and said, "When Mrs. X. asked after you the other day, I made clear to her that it was best that she not continue to see you. You've leaned on her when you have no right to her attention or resources at all." Dr. H. began to turn to walk away and then added, "More to the point, it isn't good for you!" She didn't speak to me again. Soon afterward she left on a two-week vacation and I was transferred to the care of a rotating set of residents who would simply stand at my doorway, glance in at me silently, and then move on.

The beige walls and brown spotted tile floor seemed to besiege me as I lay festering in bed. I tried distracting myself with music and television—my eyesight was becoming inconsistent, and books were proving arduous to read. By chance, two old friends from out of town visited and stayed in my new apartment. In return, they set up the furniture and unpacked a number of the boxes. One weekend evening, a friend who was a psychiatrist visited me. She asked whether she could look at my chart. I felt too ill to care that my apparent madnesses might be revealed. An hour or so later, she came back into my room and said, "They aren't doing anything for you here." She paused and then said, "A resident from gastroenterology is coming down to see you. If you haven't been moved up to that unit by Monday morning, you call me." She turned on her heels and left. The following day I was moved to a bright, modern ward in a newer wing of the hospital.

On Monday morning, a gaggle of residents and a staff physician saw me on morning rounds. That afternoon, a neurological resident came to see me. Within a few days, I had been started on a newly minted drug that increased stomach motility. Eventually, the doctors prescribed four times the recommended dose—and my stomach began to work.[2] I ate, I put on weight, and energy crept back into me. I now wanted to get back to walking. Neurology sent me for electroencephalograms and then sent me

---

2. The gastric motility drug I was prescribed was new to the market and called Prepulsid (cisapride). It was later withdrawn from general use by regulatory authorities because of the incidence of cardiac arrhythmias in individuals taking the medication.

again and again. The results for my visual EEGs caused consternation—they were abnormal when no one expected them to be. As my scalp was being wired yet again, the neuropsychologist looked at me and said, "Can I be honest with you?"

I nodded.

He bent down toward me in the gloom of the computer monitors and half-drawn blinds and said, "If I were you, I would get out of here." He straightened up slightly. "I would discharge myself," his head shook slightly, "because no good is going to come of this."

I didn't know how or what to respond. But his warning floated through my head all the rest of the day and the next. I asked to be discharged within the week. Even though I was not yet walking well, I decided that I would gain my strength on my own at home. By Friday, the staff gastroenterologist had signed my prescriptions and advised me to keep lentils out of my diet. A neurology resident stopped in. He declared that the neuro team had all agreed that I should renew my psychotherapy with Dr. D.— that my best route to health would be through his ministrations.

Despite misgivings, I called Dr. D.'s office several times—he didn't return my phone calls. When I finally spoke to him, our exchange was terse and difficult. A few years later, I learned that he had fled the local area because of pending charges of professional misconduct.

Living by myself in a downtown apartment made me feel quite grown up. I also felt isolated and lonely. The flat itself was quite pleasant: one bedroom with a small westward-facing study. The parquet floor, large doorways, and expansive bathroom meant that I could navigate it with ease in my wheelchair. The small kitchen had a lowered counter, wall oven, and separate stove top so that, in principle, cooking from a seated position was also possible. But most days I lacked the physical and psychological energy to cook for myself. I tended to eat pre-prepared meals that I heated up.

My housemates from my previous life all but disappeared. They came once or twice to visit. During one of these visits, one woman declared that she found the accessible features of my bathroom (i.e., grab bars and a raised toilet seat) so off-putting that she couldn't use the facilities. The others grabbed each other's arms, grimacing and laughing as she drew their attention to these oddities. It was the last time they visited.

Other friends were much kinder. One couple made an effort to take me grocery shopping every few weeks at one of the larger food stores. Another young woman, Abby, slept over every Thursday night. We ate dinner together and watched our favorite television shows. She always tidied the odds and ends I had left out or did a quick mop of my floor. No matter how ill or weak I felt or how irritable I became from the chronic pain that gnawed at my muscles and joints, I looked forward to her companionship. She seemed to accept me as I was—with my faults abundantly evident.

Scholastically, even as I found myself restlessly ranging my apartment, I managed to study for my doctoral comprehensive exams and passed them. The enormous and elephantine task of my dissertation lay before me. I tried to sit up at my desk to write every day, but I grew tired very easily. I found that reclining on my couch or bed most of the day left me with small bursts of energy to go outside, to read, or to work. But, nonetheless, an overall sense of exhaustion and pain dominated my days.

The abstracted and amorphous nature of my illness and disability riled me. Was I mad? I didn't feel mad. But maybe I was so mad that I couldn't recognize the reality that I was insane. But the notion of insanity and hysteria did not sit well with me. It did not have the ring of truth. Nonetheless, I fretted about my symptoms and their meaning. The uncertainty of the diagnosis along with the doctors' insistence that my poor health was my own fault made me distrust myself. Did I even know what was true or what was real? Would it ever be possible for me to have an amorous and spousal relationship with someone, especially when I couldn't control my basic physical functioning? Doubts beat their way through me in an irregular but constant rhythm. My misgivings about myself kept me from people and made me feel as though all my relationships were at some level untrue because my true self was either mad and therefore unlovable or I was so physically ill with some unknown and incurable ailment that I was not worth the effort of knowing. Despite my superficial good nature, this torturous dichotomy undercut all of my interactions.

On occasion I would have bursts of energy in which I explored the neighborhood in my wheelchair. Inevitably, even as these roamings depleted me physically, they soothed me psychologically. At home, I began to try to ride a stationary bicycle, to stand, and to take steps. Oddly, on some days these feats were possible and on others I remained too weak and enervated to even sit up in a chair. This inconstancy puzzled and worried me—the bogeyman of my own madness always haunted me, and my body's uneven performance disquieted even the most self-assured parts of myself. I did not want to be a fraud.

Even without my physical problems, I found it very difficult to concentrate on the writing that lay before me. I wasted hours watching television and listening to music. I could not take on a substantial, legitimate, and intellectualized critique of medical practice without psychologically coming to terms with my own failures and my, apparently, imaginary illness.

10 *Fire! Fire!*

In an effort to make myself feel more independent, I took physical risks that, in hindsight, I should not perhaps have taken. Moreover, despite my best efforts, I could not avoid feeling frustrated and ashamed by my condition.

An ancient parable of hysteria recounts the story of a young emir who seemed to be paralyzed. The attending physician, after much deliberation, believed the man to be perfectly healthy. One day, while he was visiting, he instructed a servant to come running into the room shouting "Fire! Fire!" In an effort to save himself, the emir jumped up and ran out of the house. In retrospect, my own courting of difficult situations was an attempt to place myself in harm's way, so that I too might be forced to leap up and cure myself. Unfortunately, one of these incidents had drastic consequences.

While living alone in my accessible apartment downtown I became friends with a woman who owned a poster and print shop. Displays of early North American maps and prints of aboriginal people enticed me into her store on a regular basis. I could look at their depictions and easily imagine a seventeenth- or eighteenth-century cartographer bent over his papers trying to capture the emerging coastlines of the Great Lakes or the Atlantic and Pacific oceans. One day the owner of the print shop invited me to join her and her boyfriend to camp at Lake Huron for a few days. I was thrilled and assured her that I could manage the rough terrain with the help of an "off-road" wheelchair. I would use it most of the time but would also rely on the fact that I could walk short distances and step over barriers that might otherwise seem insurmountable. I reveled in the prospect of fresh air, campfires, and swimming in open water.

Despite a hot and humid week at work, the weekend itself was overcast and hazy. We camped in a remote, partially cleared wood-lot acreage near the Huron shore, sleeping in separate tents and cooking over an open fire. Every few hours the skies drenched us with a fine mist. The ground was sodden. I spent a lot of time in rain gear, dragging myself across slick black logs. We lay in our tents reading, waiting for the sun to break through so that we could swim. Late on the second day, the air was warm enough that we got into bathing suits and headed to the rocky ledges at the lake's edge. Getting in was difficult and uncomfortable, the shale cut into me as I bumped my way first down and then out into the waves. But I was thrilled to be in water. Water's weightlessness always seemed like an immense relief after the labored struggle that I experienced on land. We played around for a little while and then my friends retreated back to the shore. As they collected pails of water I offered to fill a small water bottle that they couldn't carry. I lingered in the water until I realized that it was getting cold. I made my way to the shore and lifted myself slowly up the short embankment to retrieve the bottle. As I did this, it began to rain again. The rocks became slippery and uncomfortable. I decided to try to reach down to fill the water bottle rather than submerge myself again. As I stretched awkwardly below me, either my weak legs and torso gave way or I slipped. I plunged headfirst into the choppy waves. My head hit the shale bottom hard. At the same moment, I felt an extraordinary flash of fire burst in my neck and arms. Submerged upside down, I tried to bring my arms underneath me even as they seemed to be alight with flames. They were unresponsive. In fact, my whole body felt disconnected from my commands. I sloshed underneath the water. The pain in my arms preoccupied me. But then a need for air made me try to move. This time my arms did seem to drift forward. I commanded them again. They obeyed, and I lifted my head above the surf. Within a few minutes, I half knelt, half sat on the rocky bottom. I did not feel right. The rain fell on my face and the water churned around my upper chest as I contemplated my options. As it was, I felt like a misfit during this trip. I could cope, but my physical weakness embarrassed me and the foul weather of the last days made my efforts seem that much more muddy and awkward. Despite the pain and odd disconnect I felt, I decided that I would have to just slowly drag myself up the shale ledges to my off-road wheelchair. I doubted that even if I called for help—*the last thing I wanted to do was to call for help*—my friends would hear me in the darkening, rainy, and increasingly windy afternoon. After many tears and much swearing, I managed to scale the small embankment. The evening had settled in by this point, and I slid into the seat of my chair, my body and bathing suit slick with rain and lake water. By the time I propelled myself the fifty yards to the campsite, all I could think of was the Tylenol 1 pills—with codeine and caffeine— in the backpack inside my tent.[1] One of my friends unzipped the door- way to their tent and called out to me, "It's too wet for a fire; we left you a sandwich inside the cooler over there. We're going to bed."

"Sounds good to me. I think I'll do the same," I tried to offer back good-naturedly. The pain in my chest, neck, head, and arms was so in- tense I couldn't imagine eating. I fell into my tent. I immediately chewed five Tylenol 1 tablets. I then spent seemingly long, long, long minutes removing my wet bathing suit. Eventually, I lay half naked on my sleep- ing mat staring at the rain drizzling down the tent above me. I waited thirty minutes. The pain was still sickening. I reached for more tablets. I chewed another small handful. (I had no idea that I might be killing my liver by overdosing it with acetaminophen. Even if I had, I doubt I would have stopped myself. The pain was extraordinary and reached beyond my reason.) The night seemed interminable. I cried silently for much of it, muttering streams of abuse into the dank air. I lay chewing tablet af- ter tablet of Tylenol—they tasted acrid—but after about the fifteenth pill

1. This is available as an over-the-counter medication in Canada. It is not in the United States.

I felt some relief. I tried to distract myself by reading the *New Yorker* I had brought with me, but my arms were too weak to hold it above me.

Eventually, the grey light of dawn glared through the cloth walls. The rain persisted. My compatriots made movements around seven thirty. We were all miserable. They were damp and bored. I was in silent agony. Our trip to the country was fast becoming one we wanted to escape from and forget. Within the hour, we decided to pack up and drive back to the city. I suspect that we all fantasized about a hot shower. We all imagined that a bit of urban comfort might salvage the long weekend. As they packed up, I dressed. I gave up on dragging myself to the "privy" area and simply tried to pee outside my tent before taking it down. Even the act of urinating seemed tenuous, though I managed to expel something out of my bladder.

On the car ride into the city, I chewed still more tablets. I had never experienced such debilitating and unremitting pain. I wanted to scream and moan out loud. Instead, I consciously muffled myself. My headstrong silence must have made me seem bad tempered and morose. I felt too awful to make pleasantries. When they dropped me off outside my apartment building, we were all relieved to part.

Home at last, relief rushed through me at my anonymity and invisibility. I sat in the bottom of a warm shower with water cascading over my shoulders. I could now weep and blubber aloud without the risk of anyone hearing me.

I crunched yet more Tylenol and blubbered through another night, this time with a television to distract me. I didn't want to go near a doctor or hospital. No one ever knew what was wrong with me, and no one ever seemed to believe me. I made a plan to see a physiotherapist at the sports medicine clinic I had used as a university athlete. Recently, I had returned to using it in an effort to make myself more fit. I imagined that I needed some sort of neck adjustment and the pain would suddenly melt away and all would be well.

I could no longer stand, and transferring to my wheelchair required much more effort than usual.

The next morning, I took a taxi to the clinic. When I wheeled in, James, my physio, looked at me with concern, "Man, you look awful!"

"Yeah, I feel awful. I did something to my neck this weekend."

He queried me a bit more. I felt stupid, but I briefly explained my un-gainly fall into the lake. "Look, I am in agony, I was wondering whether you could do something for me?"

"Let me look at you a bit more. Hold out your arms. Open up your hands. Is that all you can do? Last week your hands worked fine."

He was right. My fingers looked clawlike, and I couldn't straighten them fully.

He expelled a breath between his teeth, "Jesus."

"What?"

"I'm going to get some help, but I think we need to get you into a neck collar."

His words frightened me. "Really? Don't you think that's a bit over the top?"

Within a few minutes he and the clinic physician, Dr. J., slipped me into a neck brace and lifted me onto a plinth. After examining me a bit more, James concluded that my legs were weaker and more spastic than the previous week. With urgent looks on their faces, they told me I needed to go to the hospital immediately.

I met their concern with anxious denials, "Look it can't be that bad? I *really hate* hospitals. *I hate them.*" I spoke with emphasis. "If you can give me painkillers, I'll just go home and sleep it off."

They looked grave and shook their heads. "In fact we've already called for an ambulance to take you."

"No," I thought, "I don't want this." I was in terrible pain, and my functioning was diminishing, but now, in spite of all my prior capacities, hospitals had become places of suffering, regret, and rebuff for me. My experiences as a patient meant that any form of medicalization seriously threatened me. I was afraid of my symptoms—at some level I now under-stood that they were serious—but if I could have somehow looked after them by returning home and importing whatever treatment or assistance I needed, I would have done it instantly.

A short while later I found myself lying prostrate on a spinal board and encased in a plastic cervical collar in an emergency unit downtown.

James and Dr. J. had accompanied me and were now speaking to a couple of trauma physicians somewhere behind my head. After a few more minutes, they tapped me on the shoulder, bent down over me briefly and wished me well. They disappeared behind a swish of curtains and were gone. I felt utterly alone.

Amid my confusion and anxiety I hoped simultaneously for two things: that the physicians would actually find something wrong with me and that it would be both treatable and relatively minor. The possibility that they would find nothing wrong seemed very likely. But I was not sure I could psychologically endure this nondiagnosis. The pain was far too intense for me to believe that it arose from my mind, that it was all a fabrication of an unstable personality.

Within moments, a nurse and resident began to undress and examine me. They asked me to tell them what brought me there. I told them the story of my lakeside fall. Another physician appeared. Again, I recounted my story. He asked me to hold out my arms, grab his fingers, bend my legs, and wiggle my toes. I obeyed his commands. His reflex hammer banged at various parts of me. He asked me to tell him when he pricked me with something that looked like a hat pin. I felt the sharpness on the insides of my legs and then up around my collarbone and neck and face. Though the feeling in my face had never equalized since a previous bout of weakness a few years earlier, I didn't want to conflate the situation, so I simply lied that the pin felt as sharp on one cheek as it did on the other. I had lived with perceptual imbalance in my face for years, and frankly I hardly noticed it anymore. I concluded that it was circumstantially irrelevant. The huddle of faces above me now moved off to one side. Two minutes later, the resident returned, "We're going to send you for a CT scan. We need to rule out a spinal injury. We're also going to have you do something called an extension X-ray. We'll remove the collar for that and then put it back on—at least until we have a better idea of what is going on." He paused, "Any questions?"

I had innumerable questions, but they all seemed locked in my throat. "No," I simply responded.

"Do you have anyone who you would like us to call?"

"Not at the moment." I couldn't even begin to think of anyone. I didn't want to call on anyone unless absolutely necessary.

The extension X-ray unnerved me. I should perhaps have been more concerned about the faded strength in my body and the increased difficulty I had moving around. But I had coped with fluctuating weakness and paralysis for years, and I'd tried to become inured to the vicissitudes of my body by adapting to changes as they occurred. I just wanted to get on with whatever task confronted me. I had lost my ability to bear weight before and had always gotten it back, so my increased immobility didn't spark too much alarm. But when the technician and resident asked me to bend my head back as far as it would go and I discovered that my skull rested heavily on my back and that I almost literally had eyes in the back of my head, I felt increasingly anxious. I held this position as they took the X-rays. When I was asked to straighten up, I couldn't. So, I hastily grabbed at a tuft of hair on my forehead and pulled my head upright.

A few minutes later, I once again lay encased in the cervical collar. I stared at the ceiling tiles and determined that I would ask for pain medication the next time I saw someone. My capacity to suppress the fire that enveloped me was diminishing rapidly. I didn't want to scream or cry, but my dignity was crumbling; tears occasionally dribbled down the sides of my face.

Suddenly, the resident loomed above me, "Well, I'm sorry to tell you this, but you've broken your neck."

My stomach fell away, as I felt suspended by an intense sense of weightless disbelief. "You're kidding me. Right?"

"No. The CT scan looked okay. But the extension X-ray shows a hypermobility of the c-spine. You've got a soft-tissue injury which allows C4, C5, and C6 to slide out of place."

I struggled to follow his reasoning. "But no broken bones, no broken neck, right?"

"No. It's good you have no broken vertebrae, but you've bruised your spinal cord nonetheless because you've torn ligaments at the front of your neck." He tapped my head lightly, "We're leaving that collar on now.

You're going to be admitted. And neurology and neurosurgery are coming to see you." He motioned to a figure beyond my gaze, "Make sure you put another sandbag beside her head."

I had been in hospitals enough and seen spinal cord patients from a distance in rehab to know that his words now placed me in a terrible situation. A breathless shock engulfed me. I could only concentrate on the details, "Could I have something for the pain?"

"Yup. I'll get the nurse to give you a shot. You're not allergic to codeine are you?"

"No."

"Now. We should also call your family."

Damn. I had worn through so many friendships in the last few years—and I knew it. Who the hell was I going to call? The choices were not happy ones. Whomever I called would once again be witness to the disaster of my life. I stumbled a little and finally blurted out the name of an academic colleague as well as an old friend of my parents who had reliably shown up whenever I summoned.

The next morning, a gaggle of doctors gathered around the foot of my bed. Lying flat and immobile, I couldn't make eye contact with any of them. They chatted among themselves. Finally, an older man broke away from the group, pulled back my blankets and asked me to move my legs, bend my arms, and grasp his fingers. He asked a young woman to assess my reflexes. She pulled out a plastic dowel with a red rubber disk on the end from the buttonhole of her short white coat. She moved around the bed, her hands trembling with nervousness. She picked up one of my legs uncertainly, glancing at one of her colleagues for guidance, "I hold it like this, right?" He reached over and adjusted her grip.

As she laboriously worked her way around my body, being corrected, chastened, and then praised, I wanted to disappear. Finally, the older physician turned to me and said, "Well, we're waiting for your chart from T. hospital to come over. We've made a referral for physio and occupational therapy to see you." He scanned a small notepad in his hand. "We also may send you for an MRI. We'll have a better sense of things tomorrow." He looked back at me, "Any questions?"

I had many questions, but I was afraid of the answers so I simply said, "No."

Over the next couple of days, as I lay miserably contemplating my future, I found that once again I was not always sure of where my arms and legs were. In the morning, when I woke, I hazarded a guess about whether either leg was bent or straight. At times I felt my limbs to be in a certain pose, and when I looked, they were in quite another. This disquieted me, but I had experienced something similar when I had severe bouts of weakness before, although during some of those occasions I was comparatively more mobile. I recalled being shot out of deep sleep because I thought someone had gotten into bed with me. It turned out that my weak arm had merely fallen onto my body, and, in my slumber, I had not identified it as my own. The return of this spooky disawareness of my body simultaneously intrigued and horrified me. Intellectually, I tried to imagine what might be happening, and I continued my guessing games on waking, much as a child picks at a scab.

Emotionally, the disconnect added one more unarticulated worry to my already overanxious psyche.

On the third day, one of the neurology residents stood by my bed and said, "Well, we finally got your chart from T. hospital."

"And?"

"Well, given your history, we've decided you haven't hurt your spinal cord. You haven't broken your neck."

"Oh."

"There were some inconsistencies in your physical exam anyway." He paused. "And it didn't make sense that you would wait so long after you fell to get medical help. There's no way someone with a real spinal injury would do that."

"What about my symptoms and the pain?"

"I don't know." He glared at me, "You tell me."

"What do you mean?" My insides scrambled themselves as I tried to remain coherent. "What about the extension X-ray?"

He glared at me. "We've decided that you're abnormally flexible. Most people's necks don't do that, but contortionists' do."

"But I am not a contortionist," I protested. "And I've never been *that* flexible." I tried to explain how my head had lolled unnaturally on my back during the test.

"Look. It's not my business."

"What about the MRI?"

"They're not going to bother with that now. I suspect they'll take that collar off and send you home." He dug his hands into his coat pockets and walked quickly away.

Once again, I was not to be believed. When I was younger, I calmed myself by engaging in physical exertion—climbing trees, riding a bike, hitting a tennis ball, or swimming endlessly. But my weakness imprisoned me. I lay there hating my mysterious incapacity and hating those who found both me and my body unfathomable. Unable to jump up and run, what would become of me now?

Perhaps I really was mad. And what a terrible madness to have if it were true. But the very core of my being did not believe that these symptoms were psychologically fabricated. Nonetheless, how could I not doubt myself given all the doubt around me? I was aware that while certain symptoms remained constant, such as the closed-fist pose of my hands, my overall immobility tended to fluctuate. At times, I even found it difficult to breathe, though in an effort not to appear dramatic, I kept this to myself. The fact that my inhalation and exhalation seemed fine at other times only justified this silence. In an effort to calm myself, I tried to meditate, but this only settled me for short moments.

During the next day or so, I waited pensively, unsure of both myself and those who cared for me. Each morning, a gaggle of neurology attending physicians, residents, and interns paused outside my door but didn't enter. Part of me strained to catch tendrils of their conversation; the other part of me wanted to close my eyes, cover my ears, and babble incoherently so that I could drown them out much as a small child does in the middle of a tantrum. One day they entered and told me that as I already lived in an accessible apartment, they were sending me home to await admission to a local spinal cord rehabilitation hospital.

Armed with a prescription for Tylenol 4s, a neck collar that I was assured I did not really need but that seemed to provide some protection from firestorms of pain, and a confused understanding of my diagnosis and/or prognosis, I returned to my life as a graduate student. Books and articles cluttered my desk, but my hands and arms were so weak that it made turning pages or holding a pen arduous work. My fingers functioned like awkward claws, and my arms seemed to be withering and aching away. I continued to wear the plastic collar despite feeling like a caricature of a whiplash victim. I quite literally chewed analgesic tablets every four hours to try to stop the pain. Unable to pursue my own research with any real clarity, I focused on my classes tutoring undergraduates.

I also decided to maintain a commitment I had made months earlier to participate in a conference on health-care delivery—anything to distract myself from the wretchedness of my life. A bioethics professor and friend had suggested me to one of the organizers, a woman who ran a rehab department at one of the city's more prestigious geriatric facilities. We arranged to meet at my apartment for a midafternoon lunch in September.

Even now, the memory of our meeting remains strong. Aruna wafted into my flat with a black cape thrown dramatically about her shoulders. An asymmetrical haircut and mismatched earrings framed her face. She smiled, tilted her head, and clasped my hands warmly. As we talked, sunlight refracted off the glass office buildings across the street, filtering into my small study and living room.

We quickly covered the upcoming conference. I would be the "patient voice" on a panel otherwise composed of hospital administrators and professionals. Our audience would consist of health professionals and managers from various jurisdictions. Given my increased immobility, Aruna offered to pick me up and drive me home before and after the session. As an occupational therapist, she saw little problem in the prospect of transferring me in and out of her car and into my wheelchair.

She then spoke enthusiastically of her latest project: obtaining a graduate degree in education, focusing on philosophy. She queried me closely. The friend who had introduced us, the bioethics professor, had assured her that I would be able to answer all of her questions and placate any niggling worries. Years before, a fellow graduate student, a classics scholar, had given me a piece of advice about graduate school early on, which I now passed on to Aruna: "Bs are bad. Don't get anything but As. A+ means the essay might be publishable. An A means that it is good. And an A− means that it is acceptable, but don't hand in this type of mediocre work again." If I hadn't learned this in the first weeks of my own career, I might have allowed myself to coast through an assignment or two with grades I thought were acceptable but which were absolutely not.

She suddenly looked worried, "But you don't understand, I never was the greatest student!"

"It'll be okay. Graduate school is different. In some ways it is easier to do well because you're allowed to investigate things at a depth and detail that facilitate your understanding and stimulates your thought." I paused to see if my words eased her concern. "And you will also be able to draw on help from people you know at the university." I laughed mildly, "And, now of course, you know me—another person to call!"

The conference went well, and afterward Aruna and I steadily became friends. We spoke often on the telephone. Newly divorced, she struggled at maintaining both her job and being a mother of two young children amid a complex and bitter joint-custody arrangement. In Aruna, I finally found someone to whom I could confess the true extent of my illness and, more important, the horrible questions it raised about my sanity. We had empathy for each other. For me, the emotional landscape of my childhood seemed both recent and poignant enough to offer her insight about her own children. And, as a health-care professional, Aruna could both understand my symptoms and problems as well as the implications of having a psychosomatic diagnosis. But even as we deliberated serious topics, we also found a simple comfort in each other.

One evening, with her children safely tucked in at their father's for the night, she and I decided to have dinner and perhaps watch a video at my apartment. Despite being in constant pain, I did my best to distract myself with an array of activities, and pursuing a social life was one of these. Just days before I had to go to the local hospital to have myself catheterized because I hadn't been able to urinate for several hours. So, despite the fact that I did not feel that well, Aruna and I met as planned. It would be a night that would irrevocably transform our lives. We cooked together in my small kitchen. I was too tired to eat much and moved to the couch. While Aruna finished her supper, I began to listen more than speak.

Around nine, my close friend, Abby, who came every week to spend the night, arrived. Abby had been stalwart during the previous four to five years of my illness. She possessed a sturdy sense of herself that was neither threatened nor dislodged by my frailties and narcissistic demands. I leaned on our friendship both emotionally and practically: along with her goodwill she often carried out errands for me and brought shopping with her when she came. Every week I had a companion to eat or simply watch TV with—it was a date I looked forward to. As my relationship with Aruna grew, Abby understandably became curious and we decided that it would be fun for all of us to meet. And, during that first evening, we all got on well.

But even as we chatted together, I knew I needed to lie down. Both women helped me onto my bed. Propped up by various pillows, we sipped cups of tea and listened to music from the living room. But the bed didn't help. I became more exhausted. My chest seemed rigid. I didn't want to cause myself or Abby or Aruna alarm so I just tried to breathe more deeply and regularly. My eyesight grew blurry and my perspective narrowed so that I could no longer follow the conversation. Aruna commented that I didn't look well.

"W .. e .. ll," I enunciated slowly and quietly, AI .. I .. find it .. haaard to breath-th-the." Even speaking those few words exhausted me.

Aruna stood up and with a few quick gestures tucked another pillow behind me. "There," she said, "Does that help?"

I smiled. I wanted to feel better.

Abby tried to be cheerful, "I'm just going to refill the cups. More tea?"

"Sure. Yes, that would be good. Milk and sugar in mine."

Aruna sat back down, "Here let me help you sit up." She nudged in beside me, putting an arm around me and straightening me up. "Now just relax."

"O-kay."

Abby returned with a small tray of mugs and a plate of cookies: "A little sugar might help too." She grimaced, and then looked at Aruna, "Look, I've seen her look bad before. It's just how it is. She'll be fine."

Aruna's grip on me seemed to work. We settled back as I listened to the two of them talk. Their voices undulated in the background as I slowly realized that I was not feeling better. Internally, I castigated myself for not inhaling more deeply and more often. My rib cage seemed numb and inflexible. Gradually, my visual focus contracted so that I could only see the green-and-white pattern of the bedspread.

Suddenly, Aruna's face planted itself in front of my gaze. "Look at me!" She said sharply, "Now! Breathe!" She pulled at my shoulders, heaving me more upright. "Now try harder! You need to concentrate." I sensed panic in her. "Breathe deeply! Try again!" She was almost shouting at me.

I tried to refocus, but it was as if all energy and movement were being sucked out of me.

Aruna now threatened me, "If you don't get better, we're going to have to call 911!" This ultimatum shot adrenaline through me, and my lungs opened up. During the past weeks we had spoken of my illusory illness and its progression. Although my symptoms had largely been written off as psychological, ironically, I had also been warned that a cervical injury was also still a real possibility (which is why I had been referred to a spinal rehab hospital) and that I needed to watch for worsening paralysis. I vaguely wondered whether I was now experiencing this. And, if so, would the solution to my problems be something I did not want and could not endure? Aruna was acutely aware of my worries. In the hospital I was totally dependent on people who thought my illness was a manipulation and an unconscious manifestation of a longing for affection. To them, I wasn't really ill—it only seemed as though I was ill. Calling 911 was the last thing I wanted.

But my recovery was momentary. Even tapping into my deepest fears could not suppress the weakness and exhaustion that now preyed on me. Blackness was setting in, and somewhere in the background I heard sirens. Abby and Aruna had made the call.

I remember being propped up on a stretcher, oxygen hissing on my face.

In the ER, voices crashed about me. My clothes disappeared with tearing sounds. Green-clad limbs danced in front of my limited view as an IV was established and lines and monitors attached.

The emergency physician who attended me, Dr. K., knew my medical history—we knew each other by name. He had, in fact, been present when I awoke paralyzed from anesthesia three years earlier. He also knew that my spinal cord injury (and all my other ailments) were questionable. He quickly whisked me into a private area of the unit. He crouched low down beside the stretcher so that I might see him and looked up into my face, "You're going to need to be intubated. We're going to have to put you on a ventilator. It's a machine which breathes for you." He hesitated. "Do you understand?"

I understood—but I wasn't sure I wanted to be put on a ventilator. I had spent the past few years getting sicker. There were times when I seemed to improve, but they were offset by longer and deeper plunges into pain and illness. The physicians may not have known what was wrong, but I knew that I was slowly getting worse. I wasn't sure I could face more. I loathed hospitals. I feared them. I feared their pain and isolation. But mostly, I feared the clinical disbelief that accompanied my admissions.

"Now, I should tell you, if, in fact, you do have a cervical injury, there is a possibility that you may never come off the ventilator—that you may always need it."

The thought of being permanently ventilated terrified me. I mouthed, "No."

He took one of my hands in his. "You don't want to be ventilated?"

Again, I mouthed, "No."

He intoned, "I think you know that you might die without it." He paused.

"I want you to think about this? Are you sure?" He kept his eyes on me. "I don't think you should decide so quickly. You're young, remember. You should give yourself a chance—*please* don't decide yet."

My breathing was slowing, but I was still straining to inhale. I was exhausted and confused. But I was still fighting. I wanted to live.

"Do you know what you want to do?"

"No." I wasn't sure.

Dr. K. held my hand and looked intently at me, "Okay, at least let me help you?"

His tone—his words and gestures—created trust. I believed him. I felt he would look after me. "Okay," I silently responded.

"I want to move you to intensive care. But not here. I don't think they'll look after you very well here. I want to send you back to T. W. Hospital."

Part of me didn't want to go anywhere—I just wanted to go home. Another part of me wanted to live. I assented reluctantly.

"Good. Let's go!"

Once again I was rushed through city streets in the back of an ambulance. When I arrived at T. W. I was taken into a room and laid flat. I remember that a man and a woman slid their stethoscope pads across me. I couldn't speak. They put me in a hallway, then in another room.

The next thing I knew I was being bagged.[2] My eyes cleared a little and I saw people above me. I didn't want this. I didn't want to be there. I heard a voice say, "Let's intubate." A panic coursed through me. What if I didn't ever come off the ventilator? I tried to move my head away from the hands in my face.

"Don't do that!" A young woman shouted at me. "No! Don't do that!"

I shook my head again. I heard another voice say, "Maybe she doesn't want it."

The woman leaned over me again. She pressed her face towards mine, "Look, I'm Dr. L." She shouted, "Intubate or die!"

The political theorist rose up in me: Was she really offering me a choice? I wanted my options better expressed. I was afraid of the ventilator. I was afraid of doctors and hospitals. But my fear of dying was stronger. In

---

2. Bagging is a procedure in which a mask is placed over the mouth and nose of a patient. The mask is attached to a rubber balloon. When the balloon is compressed manually, air is forced into the patient's lungs.

retrospect, I offered up the thinnest form of consent possible—my desire to live simply overruled my essential distrust of those who now cared for me—and so I stopped struggling.

Instantly hands were upon me. A tube bored through my right nostril. A needle sunk into my throat. I wanted to scream. I became aware of a searing pain in my nose and throat. The tube was taped to my face. I was in agony. My being was shot through with terror and with pain. I was crying. I was in hell. I wanted to go home. I *really* wanted to go home.

Through all this I heard someone say, "She's bucking the vent—I can't get it set right." Dr. L. stood by the side of the stretcher, "You've got to stop trying to breathe. The machine does it for you. Just stop breathing."

I didn't want to stop breathing. *I didn't want to stop trying to breathe.* I wanted to go home. I didn't want to be in the hospital. If I let go, if I gave myself over to the machine it would mean that I submitted to being there. It meant that I had given up. More important, it meant that I trusted them, and I didn't.

"Okay, well let's get her up to the ICU and try another vent."

The ICU seemed to hum with machinery. Abby and Aruna stood above me. I continued to try to breathe against the vent. I couldn't stop myself. I felt desperate and inconsolable. I lay on my back encased in a neck brace. Pain seared through my arms, neck, and head, and it tore at my throat.

Nurses periodically fiddled with my tubing. I dreaded them suctioning my airway. Any grappling with the tube in my nostril brought reflexive tears.[3] After an X-ray, I was rolled onto my side. I could stare out at the wall, at the machines, and at my friends. I could move my arms a bit, and I could write barely legible notes on scraps of paper. I couldn't talk. Hours passed slowly. I didn't know whether it was day or night, the ICU seemed incessantly active and bright. Thankfully, Aruna put Walkman headphones over my ears. I clutched at the strains of music filtering

---

3. Suctioning is a procedure in which the ventilator is temporarily disengaged from the tube going into the throat and lungs. A smaller, thinner tube is inserted down into the lungs and fluid is suctioned out of the airway. Once complete, the thinner tube is removed and the ventilator is reattached.

through the earphones. My eyelids shut, and I tried to hide in the music. I drifted in and out.

Throughout this initial melee, Aruna remained by my side. She held my hand, stroked my face, and wiped my tears. Her face always hung in my view—framed by the bed rails and the various tubes emanating from me. Her presence anchored my endurance. In my five years of being ill, no one had sat with me as she did now.

A day or so later, I became conscious of nurses gossiping at the foot of the bed. They shuffled through the papers of my chart. They muttered and pointed. I tried to listen, but I could only catch fragments of words. I could guess at what they were saying. No one knew why I wasn't able to breathe. Perhaps I was putting it on. Perhaps I was faking. Perhaps I wanted attention. It was too painful to contemplate; I tried to ignore them. Another day passed, maybe it was two. I wasn't sure.

A doctor came by. She bent down and told me that there was no reason that they could find for my inability to breathe. My neck injury wasn't serious enough. She was going to turn the vent off and remove the tube from my throat. She quickly extubated me. The infernal pain of it in my nose and throat ebbed. I soared with relief that the tube was gone. But within a few seconds, I was fighting for air. I sucked at the oxygen mask hissing on my face. My breaths were slow and shallow. I felt my whole being grapple for each one. I looked up at her and saw her face fill with confused concern. "Oh," she said. "It'll take a few minutes for you to get used to being without the machine. You'll work it out." She turned to the nurse, gave her instructions, and left. I gasped on.

I maintained normal oxygen saturations with extreme effort. I felt the hostility of the medical staff as they watched me in disbelief as I struggled. Their incredulity at my agony tortured me; better to die gasping at home alone in my own bed than like this.

I began to tire. I fell asleep to nightmares of mountain climbing at too high an altitude. My head pounded as I staggered through glacial snows. I cursed myself for not bringing oxygen canisters on the final push to the summit. Fields of glinting ice sheared through my eyes and into my skull. My head hurt. I wanted to be sick.

I awoke to a nurse and doctor slapping my face over and over and shaking me. "Stop that!" Stop that!" they shouted.

I looked up at them in puzzlement. My head still pounded.

"That's better. Her saturations are back up." One of them warned a finger at me, "Don't do that. Keep breathing!"

I watched them talking to one another at the end of the bed. I looked at the ceiling. I wanted to get up and run. I wanted to cry but held myself in check. I turned the Walkman back on and drifted back to the music.

Again I was on the mountain top, feeling sick. I put one foot in front of the other. I kept climbing. I wasn't sure I would make it down. My head hurt. I couldn't see properly. The sun and snow were blinding. I sat down to hold my head in my hands. The sky swirled around me.

"Hey! Hey! Breathe!" A nurse gripped my head in her hands. I heard the wailing of an alarm nearby. My oxygen saturations had sunk to 75 percent.

I looked at her. I was trying to breathe. I thought I was breathing better—not great, but better.

"Stop holding your breath!" She lectured me. "There's nothing wrong with you."

"Just leave," I thought. "Get the hell out."

"Now keep breathing, or I'll have to get the doctor back in here!"

I scowled: I didn't want to see any more doctors or nurses. I'd had it with all of them. I wanted to be any place else but in that hospital room.

I lurched back onto the mountainside. And again back into the ICU. And back again onto the steep slope. I bounced back and forth between the glacier and the inhospitable glower of the ICU. I remember little except for the pounding in my head and the searing pain in my body.

Eventually, I was moved out of the ICU. My breathing was apparently stable. I found myself one last time on the barren mountain peak. I bent over to catch my breath and threw up on my boots.

I awoke in a wardroom with an oxygen mask against my face, vomit on my chest. I tried to roll myself over but couldn't. The call bell was by my hand. I pressed it and waited. No nurse came. My chest gradually dried.

Hours later Aruna swung through the doorway. My heart bounded to see her.

"Get a gun, and just shoot me—I want to die!"

"No, you don't. No, you don't. I'll get you cleaned up and feeling better."

"Just get a gun—I want to die!" I said. And I meant it.

11 *Love in the Midst of Ruin*

The neurosurgical unit overlooked a dilapidated but busy downtown intersection. Chain stores occupied three corners. A bramble of telephone and streetcar wires wound itself in a chaotic tumult over the heads of pedestrians and cars. From where I lay, I could hear a chorus of car horns rise up from the street when, invariably, an electric bus's or a tram's power rod would become dislodged in the melee and the transit car's inert body would obstruct three or four lanes in several directions. The driver would then get out and wrestle with two large bungeelike cords and half-haul and half-bounce the power rod back onto its groove. Only then would the cacophony of traffic dissipate. This seemed to occur at least once a day.

Aruna visited regularly. As my breathing troubles ebbed, I dogged her with questions: What did she think was wrong? Would I get better? Would I stand or walk again? What did she think? Was I crazy? Was this all in my head? We had the conversations that should have been taking place between myself and my physicians, but the early morning gaggle of clinicians seemed to sidestep my bed. When the group did stop, a stony cloud of distrust permeated the air. Our exchanges were terse.

As an occupational therapist, Aruna focused on my function and on trying to preserve and make the most of what movement I did have. The uncertainty surrounding my diagnosis did not scare her away. She neither minimized nor dramatized my troubles. What she keenly saw—and what drew me to her even more—was that I wanted to live as actively and fully as possible regardless of my frailties. That she recognized and validated this core meant that she helped me hold on to a thin strand of equanimity despite my flagging morale. We grew closer. And very gradually we began to realize that our connection was something more than friendship.

In the privacy of my single room, she kissed me one evening. We stared wordlessly at each other, bewildered. We kissed again. And again. A torrent of emotion seemed to explode with each touch of Aruna's lips. Despite her gentleness, it almost hurt to have her lips softly grazing the skin of my cheek. Even as a current passed between us I wondered what the hell I was doing. This was the last thing I needed—to love a woman—to be a lesbian. I had enough working against me. But I also knew that love was the very thing I needed. And despite internal censorship, I embraced Aruna and embraced it. In the midst of hell, trapped in a malfunctioning, agony-ridden, and paralytic body, a carnal-spiritual love had found me, and I fell gratefully into its embrace. Our initial lovemaking that night was speedy and surreptitious—it was a moment that even now I look back on with awe and delight.

I rarely talked with medical staff. Nurses were less consistent. Some rarely answered my call bell, while others were very conscientious in assisting me in positioning myself in bed and arranging items so that they remained within my reach. With my permission, Aruna met with two friends who acted as my next of kin. A young professorial couple, they possessed a benevolent but sharp intelligence that I trusted. In an effort to improve my care and galvanize my move to spinal rehab, they wrote my attending physician a letter indicating their support of me. But even as we hoped that this might place me in a better clinical light, their endeavors backfired. The staff psychiatrist who had been put on my case began to question their interest in me. He asked to meet with the woman professor. When they met, he pushed at her psychological defenses, probing her motives and reducing her to tears. Instead of lifting me up, their goodwill had led to their being sullied by association with me. This taught me that hospital staff psychologized anyone who stood with me and questioned their psychological makeup and intentions. That people came under attack just for acting as my next of kin was really disturbing. It seemed that my "not yet diagnosed" status could not only imperil me but also could denigrate those around me.

The same psychiatrist pushed at me as well. He became convinced that I had had sexual relations with my father and that my problem lay in not acknowledging such an unhealthy liaison. This would apparently rationalize my mother's disapprobation of me. I couldn't believe this had happened, but given the insistence of the "experts," I wondered, could it be true? What if I didn't know myself as well as I thought I did? Was I so deeply hysterical that I couldn't recall such events?

I distrusted the psychiatrist. But in an effort to wean him of his focus on my friends and to try to entertain his theories, I met with him several times. I also submitted to a variety of psychological tests. Consequently, I agreed to a sleep study that was intended to demonstrate that I moved limbs, during my sleep, that remained immobile during the day. But the test did not bear this out. It was deemed "unhelpful" because the electrodes attached to my legs and trunk did not register the anticipated movement.

After several weeks of no progress, a doctor visited me from the spinal rehab hospital. Dr. M. examined me carefully, speaking little. Finally, she stood back from the bed and told me that a space had opened up in her facility; but she cautioned me that I would only be accepted as a patient if my respiration remained stable. She looked at me intently, "We do not take patients who require ventilation or respiratory support. Do you understand?"

I understood. She required a promise that I would not "misbehave" again. Even though I believed that I had little or no control over such a misdeed, I promised her that I would not stop breathing.

"Good." Dr. M. picked up her bag, "You'll be transferred on Friday afternoon. I'll go write in your chart."

The grounds of the spinal cord hospital backed onto a city ravine and large public park. The hospital's manicured lawns fell away into deciduous shrubbery and copses of immature trees. On one of my first evenings,

I sighted a fox trotting just beyond the perimeter. Inside, wide doorways yawned into wide hallways. Off these corridors, the wards easily accommodated four desks and beds as well as wheelchairs and other furniture. Large windows rose almost from the floor creating unobstructed views. Accessible bathrooms accompanied each room. The ground floor housed therapy gyms and equipment, a dining room, a library, television rooms, and rooms with pool tables.

On my admission, a nurse outlined various policies. Unless confined to bed as the result of pressure sores, all patients were expected to eat in the dining room. Television sets were not available in bedrooms. Even quadriplegics were not allowed automated beds. Patients signed on to an exercise schedule (occupational and physical therapy) and were responsible for retrieving medication from nursing staff. Patients were not necessarily seen as sick but as needing to adjust to altered bodies and to relearn essential activities of independent living. The policies focused on improving and maximizing individuals' physical function. Their aim was to return even severely injured or incapacitated people to their families, communities, and jobs.

The hospital's ambiance and tone reassured me. The mystery surrounding my diagnosis receded. In this context, it seemed less relevant. My physician and therapists shared the same goal I did: for me to live as independently and fully as possible regardless of my symptoms. I hadn't felt that health-care professionals were so clearly on my side since that brief encounter in the ER with Dr. K. when he had knelt down beside me to face down the demon of my impending respiratory failure.

The presumption was that I wouldn't walk again. Rehabilitation focused on strengthening the musculature that worked, increasing the flexibility in various limbs, and acquiring skills such as bumping curbs in a wheelchair, getting up off the floor, bladder catheterization, bowel management, and transfers. Therapy sessions were tightly scheduled, and I found the pace exhausting. Gradually, because my fatigue was so great, a two-hour daily rest was added to my schedule.

Slowly, I nonetheless improved. With aggressive and constant stretching, the contractures in my legs and hands eased. During my stay in the acute-care hospital, my bladder catheterizations had only been intermittent. Eventually they were stopped altogether because psychosomatic paralyses do not affect autonomic body functions. By the time I arrived at the spinal cord hospital, one of my kidneys was infected and enlarged due to a chronic backing up of urine. Fortunately, after mastering self-catheterizations, my renal function began to recover. As well, I had developed a pressure sore that refused to heal. Dr. M. ordered me to bed. My only mode of locomotion became a wheeled "banana cart." Lying either flat on my stomach or partially on my side, I could wheel around the hospital as well as continue a limited selection of my therapy exercises. The location of the sore was such that I was positioned mainly on my side, and so this made even the banana cart an unwieldy experience. Fortunately, Aruna and her children visited almost every day, which helped to alleviate my frustration and boredom. It was almost two weeks before Dr. M. agreed to allow me to sit up for limited periods in my wheelchair—but I was utterly relieved to regain my freedom.

As I grew stronger, I theorized about the origins of my problems. Perhaps, I wondered, the hypermobility of my cervical spine was the source of all my weaknesses and paralyses. Maybe when my neck was extended for intubation and ventilation during previous surgeries, it had cut off either nerve or blood supply to key areas and this had produced the postoperative symptoms. I proposed my theory to Aruna and then to Dr. M. Rather than dismissing me, Dr. M. ordered an MRI scan and referred me to a well-known neurosurgeon.

About a week later, an ambulance picked me up in my wheelchair and transported me to a nearby hospital. After the test, as we lurched through heavy traffic, my body jerked involuntarily back and forth. Despite the cervical collar, I felt the intractable nerve pain in arms and head breach my psychological reserves. I arrived back at the rehab unit in streams of tears. Up until then, given my tenuous status as a legitimate patient, I had tried to be as compliant and inconspicuous as possible. But that day, the constant and intense agony crested so that I simply could no longer keep quiet.

Dr. M. responded quickly. But her suggestion scared me: morphine. The word conjured up images of addiction. Even in my extreme discomfort and depression I worried that I would become psychologically and physically dependent. She tried to reassure me. The hospital pharmacist came to visit me. He sat beside my bed in a short white coat, sketching out the narcotic's molecular structure. He showed me articles on the use of morphine for chronic pain. My apprehension eased as he explained that I would not "get high" nor would I necessarily become addicted as long as the morphine met my pain rather than flooded it. He warned me that the first few doses would produce nausea but that it would pass. Finally, with the pain gripping my consciousness, I relented. Dr. M. ordered an immediate change in my medication. I threw up twice that night, but the burning fire began to subside. The next day I threw up again, but by evening I was less nauseated. More important, the pain in my head and limbs receded and became background noise in the normal soundtrack of my awareness. I could now concentrate well enough to read. I could also pursue my exercises with greater vigor. Quite simply, the morphine changed my life and helped it become much more livable. Within a couple of weeks, I no longer needed the cervical collar—I wore it only to combat the to-and-fro pitching when in a vehicle.

A few weeks later, Aruna drove me to my neurosurgery appointment. The surgeon was a quiet but affable man in his forties. He examined me carefully. He had read through my chart and, despite the psychosomatic diagnosis, treated me with what appeared to be genuine concern and respect. I proposed my ideas to him and very nearly begged him to perform a surgery to "stabilize" my spine by laminating several disks together. Even as he discussed the operation, he argued that while my cervical spine was problematic, the ambiguity about the cause of my paralysis was too overwhelming—he could not undertake such a risky treatment without clear cause. Although I was desperate for a solution, I understood his qualms. Faced with uncertainty and the loss of a dim hope, Aruna and I cried in each other's arms in the basement of his building afterward. Then we drove back to the rehab hospital.

My progress was steady. Fortunately, I already had an accessible flat to live in. As I grew stronger and more stable, Aruna and I planned for my discharge. Quite quickly I mastered all of the necessary skills that I would need to live in my apartment. After much consultation with my therapists and Dr. M., we set my release date for April. So as the seasons started to turn for the better, I went home.

Through the generosity of an old friend, I also learned to drive a car with hand controls. I retook my driver's license test and passed. To resume my life as a graduate student, it was clear I would need a car. Again, my friends proved invaluable. Within a few months of leaving the hospital, they raised enough money to adapt a small van for me to use. I christened it *Libertyship*. Being able to navigate the city at will opened up my life incredibly. Even now, as I look back, I believe that there is no way I would have completed my degrees and eventually found work if I had not had that car. I tired far too easily to endure the long waits—often lasting hours—for the local handicapped transit. The little white van liberated me. It allowed me to act with a degree of autonomy that had long been removed from my life. I loved the car as a result, and I loved those who had made it possible.

Given that I was still a quadriplegic for no apparent reason, Aruna and I both presumed that the course of my illness might be downward and that I would not likely live long. Dr. M. seemed to concur with this possibility. I decided that we would go on a holiday to the seaside with what remained of my savings. I love the ocean and wanted to swim in its salty waves once more. I certainly wasn't well enough to travel alone and I entreated Aruna to go with me. After much urging, she agreed. The Americans with Disabilities Act had just been adopted in the United States and it seemed like the most reasonable destination given the statute's mandated accessibility of private and public spaces. In the end, we flew to South Carolina. I had to be carried on and off planes, and the hotel was barely accessible. With Aruna's help and an off-road wheelchair, I could get to the beach and float off my chair and into the toss of the surf.

We ate well, sketched, and read books to each other while lying in the shade of an umbrella on the sand. I convinced a tour operator to wedge me into a sea kayak and tape my hands to a paddle so that we could tour the coast. That evening we paddled among dolphins as they dined on the discards from a shrimp boat. After this venture, it was relatively easy to talk Aruna into going deep-sea fishing. We caught mahi-mahi, which were filleted and then frozen to take home. We also drove to Charleston and toured plantations. For ten days the air hung heavy with humidity and sunshine. We rested well. Aruna and I became more intimate lovers, and unwittingly this trip became our honeymoon.

Within the year (I was now twenty-six), Aruna and I and her two young children found a place to move into together. We knew our friends thought we were mad. The last thing Aruna, a newly divorced and single mother, needed was to be "looking after" a quadriplegic. The last thing an enfeebled, narcissistic cripple needed was to be moving in with young children. I was in no apparent physical shape to look after them.

Our first home was a three-story townhouse with a platform lift that carried me up the staircases in my wheelchair. While we hosted parties to celebrate our new life, we also chafed at the prospect of living as "out" lesbians. I could not even utter the word lesbian aloud. It seemed indecent, even grotesque. Fortunately, most of my friends were either academics or artists, and all of them seemed to welcome Aruna as my partner. This made acclimating to my new sexuality somewhat easier. It was difficult to loathe myself for falling in love with a person of the same gender when those around me didn't condemn me for it. Unfortunately, Aruna's health-care colleagues were less positive. One or two took her aside and cautioned her. Another was openly belligerent toward me when we had her to dinner and accused me of trying to sabotage Aruna's life and career.

Remarkably, while we all needed to adjust to one another, goodwill predominated. Aruna's two children, a son, Justin, and a daughter, Alisha, were charming. They were used to a number of adults being in their lives—from a multitude of aunts and uncles and baby-sitters to parental friends. Meeting the demands of her mortgage meant that Aruna had had roommates since divorcing, and both Justin and Alisha didn't notice a difference in my status except that Aruna and I shared the same room.

We decided not to thrust information about our sexuality on the children, but we did speak of ourselves as a couple. Gradually they realized that I was more than a roommate and that my presence was not based on financial convenience but love.

Alisha, Justin, and I discovered that we had an ease with one another. We were fortunate in that Aruna was not proprietary about her offspring. This allowed the children and I to negotiate and create an emotional space for one another without feeling that their mother might feel isolated or threatened. They, in turn, accepted my wheelchair and various physical incapacities without prejudice. In fact, they were often my greatest advocates, scouting out accessible routes to school concerts, restaurants, shops, and theaters.

I knew that in committing to Aruna I was also committing to Justin and Alisha. And while I was not a parent, per se, I was a responsible adult in their lives, and as such, I needed to try to ensure their emotional and physical well-being as best I could. Consequently, even as I was plagued by ongoing pain and fatigue, I always tried to be as "well" as possible for them. I took them to the park; played catch; coached them on riding bicycles, playing sports, and climbing trees; read stories; and tried to get to know their friends. Despite my daily exhaustion and the concomitant demands of meals, bath time, homework, playing, and bedtime stories, Justin and Alisha's love and attention gave me something indefinably and wonderfully good. Very slowly I realized that I had become a protoparent and that not only was I good at it, I loved it and I loved the children—*and* they loved me. So, even as my physical state became more and more fragile, we became more and more emotionally robust as a family.

Within two years, we moved to a more accessible three-bedroom apartment with large gracious rooms. During this period, I began to experience ongoing (rather than just intermittent) ptosis—weakness in the eyelids of both eyes that was so severe that they drooped closed much of the day. My nighttime breathing was so poor that I was desaturating when lying down and required an oxygen mask through the night and parts of the day. These changes were investigated with short hospitalizations but with little outcome. The only change was that I was now considered a palliative-care patient. Medically, I was dying without apparent cause. A nurse came to visit once or twice a week to counsel me about my impending death and to tend to periodic pressure sores. Every day an attendant came to help me bathe and dress. This activity was so enervating that on many days I spent the rest of the day lying in bed. The attendant would also do light housework before leaving me a small lunch on my bedside table—often I was far too fatigued to chew or swallow it. As the afternoon waned, I would gather my strength in order to transfer myself into my wheelchair so that I could be upright when the children came home. When I didn't have this strength, we would gather on "the island"—Aruna's and my bed—where they would do their homework or play games while we waited for their mother to come home. On some evenings the family ate picnic dinners on the island—with the floor becoming a sea full of sharks to be avoided when retrieving food, cutlery, or plates from the kitchen.

We tried to normalize my illness and loss of function as much as possible. And each child possessed their own form of elemental kindness, which made this easier. At times, I became too weak and ill to be kept at home and I ended up in hospital for days or weeks at a time, and then when a little bit stronger, I went home. Very little was offered to me except palliation in the form of pain control and oxygen.

I began to exhibit signs of arthritis with multiple joints swelling simultaneously. This made movement even more difficult, if not impossible. Dr. N., the rheumatologist, was an incredibly warm-hearted man who, when I thanked him for being so solicitous toward me, remarked that he tried to "treat every patient in the manner he would want his grandmother, mother, or daughter treated." He tested me for lupus, but again I was negative for the relevant serum antibodies. To try to reduce my discomfort Dr. N. prescribed a short-term increasing and then tapering dose of prednisone. But as the dosages climbed, I became unbearably weak—so weak that I struggled to swallow, speak, breathe, and roll over in bed.

In an effort to recover muscle strength, I stopped the steroids. Paradoxically, about a week or two later—it is now difficult to recall the precise time period—I felt wonderful. My joints were no longer swollen and my physical strength rebounded. I felt almost euphoric. It was as if the steroids had kick-started something inside of me. This brief treatment gave me a short-lived hiatus in which I frolicked with the children and made a little headway on my PhD dissertation. (Despite having a scholarship, I was now usually too weak to produce much academic work.)

Aruna has since told me that I was becoming so frail that she worried that she would awaken to a corpse lying next to her in bed. But my strength was inconsistent. On some days I could socialize with friends, read through books and journal articles, and write on my laptop in bed. On other days, it took all my physical resources to simply draw a breath in and then expel it. On these days, my chest walls seemed to be collapsing in on themselves, and the heavy, fatigued musculature of my upper torso seemed to crush my rib cage. It became very difficult for the attendant to position me so that I was comfortable. Once she tucked various pillows around me, I remained in the same pose until either Aruna or the children came home and moved me. At these times, when it felt as though my life force was draining away, I spent endless hours simply trying to exist.

As I became obviously weaker, with drooping eyelids and difficulty swallowing and breathing, I was often passed from specialist to specialist. Inevitably, the ophthalmologist, pulmonologist, or rheumatologist would conclude that my problems were neurological in origin and that they could do little to help me. But I had great difficulty finding a neurologist who would take me on because my medical chart said that my problems were psychosomatic. Unbeknownst to me, during one of my hospitalizations, one of the staff neurologists booked me for a nerve-conduction test of my genitals since he did not believe that I should have difficulty initiating bowel and bladder movements. A few weeks later, when I arrived for the test, the clinic neurologist looked at me in disbelief, "Do you know what he is asking for?"

"Something about testing my bladder?" I queried naively. "But, I don't know why they want this test because I had a bladder-function test done when I was in the rehab hospital. Maybe you can tell me what it is?"

He continued to look at the referral sheet. With it clenched in his hand, he turned away and retreated behind a row of filing cabinets to speak to his resident. I heard him say, "This is ridiculous," and then, "even barbaric!" and then his tone eased and the rest of his words became inaudible. A few minutes later he returned and perched awkwardly on a row of seats beside me in the waiting area. "Look, I've never even known anyone to request this test. I wouldn't even know how to do it. It can't and shouldn't be done."

"Oh." I remain puzzled, "So there's nothing to be done here?"

"No." He paused, "And I'll write a note to the doctor at T. W. hospital about it." He shook his head and stood up. "Okay?"

"That's it?"

He nodded.

I shook his hand and turned and wheeled down the length of the hallway to the elevator. It was only as I sat in the car afterward that I realized what the other doctor had requested. He had wanted to have nerve conduction studies done of my peritoneal region, which would have entailed administering small electrical shocks to my genitals and measuring the tissue's responses. A wave of heated shame and anger rode through me once I grasped what I had just narrowly escaped. It seemed that the referring physician had used a form of medical logic to (unconsciously?) punish me for my seeming malingering and refusal to get well. A few years later I would encounter an almost unreadable book by Jeffrey Masson, *A Dark Science,* in which he translates nineteenth-century medical texts in which doctors experimented on and inflicted similar type of punitive treatments on female patients they presumed to be sexually or psychiatrically unbalanced.

This incident taught me to be much more critical of what clinicians asked of me. Previously, I had tried to be as compliant and cooperative as possible so that professionals understood and respected the seriousness of my desire and efforts to get better. But this aborted investigation showed me that my strategy of good-natured compliance was not improving my care but indeed might actually be jeopardizing my well-being.

After watching me worsen over our first three years together, Aruna finally convinced an esteemed neurologist in the geriatric facility she worked in to see me. We both desperately wanted to find both a cause and a cure for my paralysis and lack of vigor. Throughout my illness, I maintained a guileless belief that allopathic medicine could provide an answer to the enigma that plagued me—I just had to find the right doctor.

12 *Grasping at a Diagnosis, Hoping for a Cure*

Originally, Dr. O. met with me for over an hour. He didn't perform a physical exam but simply asked me to recount the tale of my illness from the very beginning. Typical of his peers, he said little except to ask for occasional clarification about dates and symptoms. We booked another appointment for the following week. During this meeting, he examined me thoroughly but again said little. When we sat down in his office afterward he asked whether I would be willing to undergo more tests. We agreed to repeat a spinal tap, nerve-conduction tests, and an MRI. I had had all of these previously. However, he asked to do one test that I had never had or heard of before—a Tensilon test.

Unsurprisingly, the MRI was negative. The electrical tests came back negative as well. The spinal fluid again showed atypical oligloconal banding, but, while this result was abnormal, its meaning was not clear, as it did not follow the pattern for multiple sclerosis. The Tensilon test was a slightly different matter. Ironically, I returned to the clinic that had refused to conduct the genital-nerve studies. They injected a substance called Tensilon into me. And nothing apparently happened. After barely a minute, the resident and neurologist abruptly told me I could leave. I was astonished by the brevity of the encounter, and so I quickly left. I was in my car within a few seconds. But as I pulled out into traffic I caught a glimpse of myself in the rear view mirror—for the first time in many months both of my eyes were fully open! I was astounded and quickly called Aruna. She told me to call the clinic. When I called, the reception-ist told me that the doctors had "left for the day" as I had been their final appointment. They wouldn't be back until morning. I spoke to Aruna again and she encouraged me to call Dr. O. I hung up and dialed his of-fice. I left a message explaining that whatever I had been injected with had caused my eyelids to lift but that it hadn't happened in the office but a couple of minutes later in my car. I then drove home. The whole venture had exhausted me and I lay on our bed waiting for the rest of the family to come home. As I lay there Dr. O. telephoned me. He asked me whether my eyelids were still fully open. I didn't have a mirror near me on our bed but presumed (incorrectly) that they were and I said so. Dr. O. hung up after saying very little. A few minutes later, Aruna came home, and when I recounted the phone call she corrected me and told me that my eyelids were, in fact, drooping. I called Dr. O.'s office and left a message again, amending my early statement.[1] The end result was that without a physician present to witness the events, the Tensilon test was documented as negative. When I returned to Dr. O.'s office a couple of weeks later he indicated that he had suspected I might have a disease called myasthenia gravis but because both the electrical tests and the Tensilon test had been negative this diagnosis was no longer tenable. He had little idea now what might be wrong with me. He stated that there were three possibilities: (1) that I had a common presentation of an uncommon disease; (2) an uncommon presentation of a common disease; or (3) an uncommon presentation of an uncommon disease. He had suspected MG but did not know what to suggest since the tests had been negative.

Aruna and I once again felt deflated by our pursuit of answers and perhaps a cure. At the very least we hoped that a diagnosis that confirmed the physical origins of my paralysis and weakness might mean that clini-cians would treat me with more compassion. Despite Dr O.'s dismissal of myasthenia gravis as a possibility, we began to read up on the illness.

---

1. I later learned that the return of my ptosis made sense, since Tensilon rejuvenates weak muscles only temporarily (i.e., only for a few minutes).

Because Aruna worked in health care and because I was a doctoral student, we had access to the same medical databases that physicians used. The more we read, the more we became convinced that it was the most likely possibility.

Myasthenia gravis is a neuromuscular disease. In women it usually appears in young adulthood, whereas men predominate its occurrence in the over-fifty age group. We read at the time that the statistical occurrence was 1 incident per 1,000,000 population. As of the turn of this century, epidemiologists have revised their estimates to 1 per 250,000. Some neurologists believe that it might even occur more frequently but that it is overlooked or misdiagnosed, especially in the elderly where complaints of fatigue or weakness are dismissed as natural aspects of "old age." Two forms of the disease exist: ocular MG, affecting only the eyes, and generalised MG, affecting the whole body. Usually patients start out with ocular symptoms and sometimes progress to having overall weakness and fatigue. In such cases, if the symptoms become severe enough, people suffocate to death. In general, proximal rather than distal muscles are affected, that is, the muscles of the face and torso weaken first, thereby producing drooping eyelids; an expressionless face; and difficulty swallowing, breathing, walking, or raising the arms. One of the central features of the illness is that the more one uses a muscle, the weaker and less responsive it becomes.

Although it is a neuromuscular disease, it is also a disease of the immune system. An individual's antibodies attack the neural synapses, interfering with the communication between the nerves and the muscles. It is difficult to diagnose because it doesn't appear on X-rays, spinal taps, CT scans, or MRIs. Usually single-fiber EMGs—electromyograms—show that a muscle steadily weakens as a current passes repeatedly through it. Blood tests for specific antibodies can help, but there are myasthenics who are seronegative, that is, they do not test positive for the corresponding antibodies. Finally, if an individual reacts to the administration of Tensilon, then they can also be considered to have the disease.

Myasthenia gravis cannot be cured; however, it can be controlled. Treatment consists of suppressing the immune system with steroids and other drugs. As well, pyridostigmine (i.e., Tensilon, Mestinon) can be taken throughout the day to facilitate communication between nerves and muscles. Finally, myasthenics need to modify their activities so that they reduce fatigue—rest actually allows muscles to recover strength. Consequently, a patient's weakness and paralysis is variable. After sleeping and about an hour after taking Mestinon, tasks can seem relatively easy. However, at the end of the day, swallowing, talking, or walking may be laborious, and sometimes even taking Mestinon may not make much difference to enervated muscles. On occasion, those with generalized myasthenia—the disease that affects muscles all over the body and not just the face—can have a "crisis" in which the chest muscles and diaphragm weaken so they go into respiratory failure. This requires immediate intervention and the use of a ventilator to assist breathing. Doctors may resort to using plasmapheresis on these occasions. This is a plasma exchange in which the myasthenic's white blood cells are removed and replaced with donor white blood cells, thereby ridding the body of the attacking antibodies. Plasmapheresis is a complex and risky procedure that needs to be performed every day for a period of seven to ten days. Intravenous ganciclovir (IVG) can also be administered in an effort to quell rampaging antibodies.

Among many things, the muscle relaxants used during the administration of an anesthetic cause paralysis in myasthenics, and this correlated strongly with my own exposure to anesthesia and my subsequent episodes of weakness. In addition, paralysis tends to be inconsistent, and this was also true of me. My positive response to Tensilon encouraged our belief that we might finally have an answer. And so we approached my general practitioner, who as yet had only prescribed pain management and palliative measures. We explained the bizarre sequence of events surrounding the Tensilon test and convinced him to try me on the primary myasthenia drug: Mestinon. As a medication it has a short half-life in the body, lasting only about four hours. It also has nasty side effects, causing stomach upset and excessive salivation and sweating. Our logic was that it was worth a try, that I had very little to lose—my family doctor agreed.

And, the pill helped! Originally, I took it twice a day and began to feel my life force returning. On good days, I actually had energy. Consequently, my GP decided that I could take the pill every four hours. We also began to consider my taking steroids to suppress my immune system. I started on a very low dose of 1 milligram per day. We began very, very slowly so that I would not experience the severe weakness I had experienced when my rheumatologist, Dr. N., had prescribed larger, more accelerated doses—as is typical for arthritic conditions. In our reading we had discovered that people with MG often have the same response to prednisone: while it is useful in suppressing antibodies, too hefty a dose given too quickly can actually produce a myasthenic crisis.

Although the quantities were small, the drugs made a difference. I definitely had more energy, and I could sit up in my wheelchair more often. I applied to teach a course during the fall term. I felt so well that we accepted an invitation to do a reading at a friend's wedding in Montreal over the Labor Day weekend.

But, unfortunately, I overextended myself, and, after an active few days touring Montreal, I slipped into respiratory failure: I remember feeling increasingly tired and breathing becoming more difficult, but I attributed this to the extraordinary heat. Aruna looked over at me at a stoplight and realized that my color had turned gray. She tried to shake me out of it, but I was semiconscious. By the next stoplight, my lips were blue. Even now she does not know how she found a hospital in a strange city, but she did. She raced our little hatchback into the driveway of a trauma unit, yelling for help. Within seconds I was dragged from my seat by orderlies and nurses and hoisted onto a stretcher. I wasn't breathing, and my oxygen saturations had fallen precipitously. Aruna reported my condition as presumed myasthenia gravis. The ER physician reacted quickly. He intubated me and attached me to a ventilator. It was at this point that I became aware of my surroundings and of the tiled walls, swinging doors, IV poles, and elevators. A few minutes later, the hum of the ICU seemed docile and almost pastoral in comparison with the chaos of the ER.

The following day things became clearer. The ICU was on a high floor with large sunlit windows overlooking the roofs of surrounding buildings. My nurse was an affable French Canadian who spoke to me in English but soon discovered that I could understand the French being spattered around me. I responded to queries by scribbling on a notepad. By afternoon, a large IV had been attached to my chest and a round of plasmapheresis had begun. I instantly felt better and wanted the ventilator removed. I began to bounce back. And so, after persistent pleading, the staff physician finally agreed to withdraw the machine on the condition that I was willing to have it reattached if necessary. A portion of me wanted to jump down off the bed and prepare my reading for the wedding the following day. But, while movement was possible, the expended effort was too laborious. Aruna rehearsed the passages instead.

Even as my friends were reciting their vows, I received another round of plasmapheresis. Despite my self-reproach for ending up in ICU, I was also relieved that this hospitalization was running smoothly and that I was being treated sympathetically as well as efficiently. Both Aruna and I worried that when a copy of my chart arrived after the long weekend indicating my undiagnosed status, it would alter the caliber and tone of the care I was receiving. So Aruna tried to gently forewarn the attending physician and resident of my peripheral status among neurologists in Toronto.

Unfortunately, we were right. A copy of my chart arrived on Tuesday and a coolness began to penetrate our interactions with the staff. My once affable nurse now looked at me disapprovingly. Without warning, the IV line for the plasmapheresis was pulled out and I was told that I was being transferred out of ICU. In fact, they said that they would like to discharge me from the hospital completely. When I tried to engage the nurse and neurologist in conversation they inevitably responded that there was nothing wrong with me. I attempted to push at their newly tough veneer a little by encouraging them to reexamine my initial vital signs—how was it that I was not breathing or conscious when I arrived in the ER? They replied that the emergency room doctor must have made a mistake in reading the monitors. The neurologist dismissed me with a shrug of his shoulders and a protrusion of his lower lip. He turned and left my bedside.

I didn't have the energy to argue. Even speaking a little winded me. Interestingly, the nurse now noticed my exertion and pallor. She reattached an oxygen monitor as I tried again to speak to her. My saturations were low. She quickly left, returning several minutes later. She said that she had told the medical team about my poor oxygenation and had asked them to reconsider my impending transfer. But the doctors remained adamant and dismissed her concerns. She now looked at me with a mixture of regret and concern. I could see that my situation puzzled her. The chart's presumption that I was emotionally unbalanced originally aroused her suspicion, but now she began to try to assess me physically and compare it to the substance of the medical record. I sensed that she now doubted that my case was clear-cut. She asked another nurse to come in to examine me and to view the oxygen monitor. They said they would speak to the unit director, that is, the head nurse. But I had seen nurses and respiratory therapists argue on my behalf before, and I knew that little would likely come of it. Despite being part of "the team," their opinion was just that, an opinion; it carried little weight or power in the decision to treat or not to treat, to discharge or not to discharge—ultimately these powers belonged solely to physicians. About twenty minutes later, the head nurse introduced herself to me; she told me that she could try to forestall my discharge from ICU but that she thought it would probably be best that my care be sorted out in Toronto and with clinicians who knew me. In sum, she wanted to avoid the political ruckus that my ambiguous diagnostic status might cause.

At this point, all I wanted to do was to retreat to my home and to hide my deformities, both mental and physical, from their disbelief in me. I asked that they telephone Aruna and tell her simply: "The chart has arrived. I need to go home." I knew she would understand this seemingly cryptic missive. Exhausted and barely able to move, I slumped back on the head of the raised bed and waited for her rescue. As I lay there I tried to smother an urge to weep and weep and weep.

Later that day, Aruna guided my body into the front seat of the car. She had reclined it slightly, and an oxygen tank with a mask and nasal prongs lay propped in the leg space. The late summer heat burned through the windshield, as she tried to position my torso with pillows. Feeling too weak, I mutely pointed at things that hurt or bothered me. The delay seemed interminable. I just wanted to leave as quickly as possible. But I also knew that if I was not settled properly, I would fall over at the first lurch of the car into traffic. Even as my internal editor grew frustrated with my incapacity and with Aruna's interminable fussing, I also wanted to cling to her, sobbing my gratitude for the strength of her love. If I were her, I couldn't and wouldn't put up with all of this—I would have walked away long ago. It awed me that she stayed—that she endured my feebleness without the least assistance or even compassion from others. I knew that my reputation as a malingerer stigmatized her as well. Because she worked in health care, it might even discredit her considerable clinical and personal judgment.

Our eight-hour drive home was prolonged. At one point we stopped because I needed to go to the bathroom. But the exertion this required caused my breathing to falter. We said little as I slowly gasped amid the humid grasses by the side of the highway. I half-sat, half-lay hunched forward against the bottom edge of the car, with the door propped wide open. My head sometimes rested on the front passenger seat, but, while this eased the strain of holding it up, it caused my breathing to slow even more, and so I would push myself more upright. I groaned inaudibly throughout. Tens of minutes passed as we waited for me to either get better or worsen. In an effort to help me, Aruna crushed some of the Mestinon to strengthen me and added some morphine for the terrible pain in my body and joints. She slowly dribbled them into my throat with water. And then we waited—suspended in a torpid but dramatic microcosm of illness, sunshine, exhaust fumes, and humidity—with cars and trucks thundering by, rocking our vehicle.

Finally, the small crisis passed so that Aruna could now lift me back into the car. Again she deftly placed me in the seat with the oxygen hissing gently on my face. She tucked jackets, pillows, and blankets around me. And then she propped a kidney basin—which we always kept in the car—by my face. Eventually, she slid into the driver's seat and began to readjust the rearview mirrors and check the oncoming stream of vehicles in her side mirror. And we finally made it home.

And after a week or so in bed in our apartment, I gradually recovered my strength, and it was as if the collapse of the long weekend had never occurred. The most obvious outcome of all this was that our daughter, Alisha, enrolled in a French immersion school. Montreal had made her want to speak a second language.

I continued on the Mestinon and prednisone. My general practitioner and I tried to gradually increase the steroid dosage so that it was at 10 milligrams per day. By Christmas we got there. And while I still used a wheelchair and had periods of fatigue, my overall energy was much better than it had been without the drugs. Life seemed more possible.

Little did we know that I was about to have an even worse episode of paralysis and weakness from which it would take me at least a year to recover. Although I did not know it then, its ferocity would become the high-water mark of my illness—my life afterward would be fundamentally transformed.

13 The Crisis Deepens

I was thirty years old when I lifted myself from a bath on a gray February morning into my second respiratory failure in nine months. Within seconds, as my breathing became slower and shallower, I could no longer speak. Aruna managed to shift me from my wheelchair onto the bed.

"Are you okay?" She asked.

I shook my head.

"Oh shit! We're going to Emerg again, aren't we?"

I nodded.

Her face creased with worry, "You're sure? You're sure you want me to call 911?"

I looked at her. I knew exactly what she was asking. Could I bear another ICU stay, another intubation, and more arguments about what was wrong with me? Could I bear to be dismissed as I lay immobile and in agony? I had sometimes said that it would perhaps be better to die than to suffer through this again. I paused. I considered my options. Should I, I wondered, finally let myself die in our apartment, or should I throw myself on the mercy of physicians, who often believed I was hysterical, and endure tremendous pain, loss of dignity, and then perhaps die anyway? As the room went out of focus and the fibers of my body screamed for oxygen, I threw my arm out toward the phone that lay nearby. All I knew was that I wanted to live.

Within minutes I could smell the smoky presence of firemen and hear the squelching of rubber boots. I heard a man's voice ask, "She's paralyzed, right? She's willing to be resuscitated?"

My consciousness stirred as the stretcher banged its way through a hospital doorway. I became clearer with the pain of a tube tunneling into my mouth and throat. I instinctively reached to grab at it and felt my arms pinned to the mattress. I could feel a needle seeking an artery in my wrist again and again and again.

"Damn, I can't get it!" A young intern ceded the vial to a burly resident.

The sharp point probed again. I wanted to wrench my arm away but he held it firmly, almost painfully with his forefinger and thumb: "This isn't any good. I'm going to try the other side."

Reflexively, I tried to draw my other arm away from him. I discovered that it no longer moved. Unaware of this, he threw his weight painfully on top of my wrist. "Look," he said, "I know this hurts, but I've gotta get blood gases." He spoke to me with apologetic grimness: "We really have to know your oxygen and CO_2 levels." I counted perhaps ten tries. My eyes watered, and tears seeped through my eyelids.

"Okay. Okay," he relented. "We'll stop for the moment and try later."

The hard plastic of the tube rasped against my raw throat. My torso seemed to torque painfully around it.

A green-clad woman hovered by the ventilator. She said, "Try to stop breathing. Don't work against the vent! Just let it do it for you."

Quietly, the contents of my stomach floated up my throat and around the breathing tube and poured out my mouth and nose. It happened again a few seconds later. And then again and again every few minutes over the next several hours. It seemed as though my body was trying to eject every last piece of foreign matter. Another plastic tube was inserted in my nose and down into my stomach. Pink and black bile flowed up it and into a jar.

Soon I could no longer bite down on the tube between my teeth. My jaw was becoming slack, and saliva began to spill over my lips. I couldn't shut my mouth.

A catheter was inserted in my bladder, and a new IV was started in my right elbow. I could feel a cold stinging sensation in my forearm where the last line had blown. As I faded in and out of consciousness, people seemed to be always standing above me. Carts and machines clattered and banged as I felt the paralysis settle deeper and deeper. I began to feel like an inert, jellified custard.

My muscles felt as though they were trembling minutely and uncontrollably, although I could see they were quite flaccid. I felt as though I were caught in a rushing torrent of energy that could find no physical expression. It was as if my whole nerve and muscular system was vibrating so intensely that it became static. The sensation was not painful in any traditional sense, but it nonetheless created a barely tolerable physical and psychological agitation.

With enormous effort, I could roll the heel of my left hand back and forth and flex the fingers weakly. With a pen held loosely in my slackened fist I scrawled "*PAIN*" on a scrap of paper.

The nurse took the message into her hand. "I know, I know," she patted my arm. "First, we've got to get you to ICU."

Twelve hours later, I still lay on the stretcher in the trauma unit. I heard arguments about a lack of ICU beds.

A respiratory therapist complained, "I've got patients upstairs. Look, I can't leave her. But, for God's sake, find someone else!"

Amid the administrative chaos, my body continued to pulse out bile while simultaneously refusing to breathe with any regularity.

Finally, the staff found an ICU bed at a hospital a few blocks away. I was hooked to a transportable ventilator and lifted into a waiting ambulance. A paramedic, a nurse, a neurology resident, and a respiratory therapist all crouched in beside me.

I arrived in the early hours of morning to an amber-lit, peacefully throbbing ICU. As the admitting nurse flipped through papers by my bed, I heard her sigh, "Oh, another dump from T. hospital."

I wasn't too paralyzed to be furious. With the pen resting inside my left palm, I scratched on a pad of paper lying under my hand: "*I AM NOT A DUMP.*"

She crimsoned a little. "I'm sorry. That's not what I meant," she said. She fumbled with the chart a bit more and then picked at the NG tube that still drained pink and black bile. "Did you take something? It says here that you might be a suicide."

Christ, again? No, I signaled.

"They don't know why you're draining so much....Well, your tox screen is negative."

I scrawled "*PAIN*" on the piece of paper.

"I know, I know," she said. She looked across the room thoughtfully. "I don't know whether they're going to keep you intubated. We'll have to wait and see." She turned back to me, "So they don't know what's wrong with you, eh? It says here maybe myasthenia, but then they also want psychiatry to see you....Well, we'll get you settled. I'll get orders. And then, maybe you can rest. The neurology resident won't be up for a couple more hours."

During the next twenty-four hours, clinicians gathered at my bedside. They murmured inaudibly to one another, flipping through chart material and staring glumly at the various monitors. One of them finally addressed me, "I think we'll try to extubate you and see how it goes."

Despite saving my life, the tube and ventilator were my enemy. They inflicted intolerable pain, and I welcomed their absence. I discovered that with great concentration and effort, I could breathe on my own. But every breath strained me. My lungs worked more slowly and shallowly than I wished. But I thought I could sustain myself. My mood grew lighter.

A resident attempted to retrieve blood gases from my wrists and failed once again. Without active muscles in my face and throat, I mutely endured his prodding until I finally wrote on the pad of paper with my left hand "NO".

"All right, all right. You're pretty bruised." He stopped.

As the day wore on, I grew tired but was too afraid to sleep. I felt that if I slept, I wouldn't breathe. I feared dying. I feared resuscitation. I feared the ventilator. I chose to breathe and didn't sleep.

Into the evening, my chest began to ache. My body felt as though it were running at an accelerated pace. I tried to meditate, but my chest continued to grab at me painfully. I focused on each breath, coaching my-self to draw more deeply and with greater frequency. My body wouldn't obey. I felt ceaselessly tired and afraid.

A pale doctor appeared over me in the early hours of morning. "Are you having any pain?" he asked.

I signaled "Yes."

"Can you tell me where?"

I tried to speak, but couldn't.

"Legs?" He paused. "Arms?" He paused again. "Head? Chest?"

I signaled "Yes."

"I thought so." He rubbed his unshaven cheek. "I think we're going to try you on nitro. It's for your heart. I want you to tell me if the pain gets better, worse, or stays the same, okay?"

The pain eased temporarily.

"Okay. We'll start you on a nitro patch and a morphine drip," he patted my bedrail. "I'll see you in a few hours, I'm going to get some shut-eye."

In the morning, my bed was moved to a crowded ward in the ICU. In the corner, a young semiconscious man moaned. His father mopped his fore-head with a towel. At times, the patient's torso would twist upward and his eyes and mouth would jerk wide open. Alarms would scream and a ripple of chaos would erupt as his body broke free of various lines and machines.

Opposite me, an older woman wanted food. I could hear her plead-ing for something to eat: "I'm *so* hungry! I haven't eaten since yesterday morning! Please give me something to eat. I'll even take Jell–O." Her nurse was circumspect: "Not yet. Maybe in a couple of days." I overheard the staff physician tell someone that she was in liver failure. Surgery had revealed a large tumor elsewhere as well. "When you get to the floor, may-be they'll let you eat then," her nurse consoled her.

Later the same day, a female psychiatrist stood by my bed. "You don't look so good," she commented. She looked around the room. "God, don't you want to get out of here?"

The question stabbed at me.

"Look, I don't think there's much I can do here. They think you might have taken something." She looked down at the binder wedged in the crook of her arm. "I don't get it. Your tox screen's negative." She looked back at me questioningly, "So, did you take anything? Did you try to off yourself?" She paused for my answer. "No? Good." She wrote something down. "To be frank, I don't know what I can do. Do you need anything?"

I needed to breathe. I needed to move. I needed to be anywhere but there. I signaled "No."

"You don't look like you need me. You look like you need a neurologist.... It's okay if I don't come back?"

In the afternoon, Aruna was holding my hand when two residents appeared at my bedside. Soon an older physician, Dr. P., arrived along with some medical students. The head ICU nurse introduced herself and perched on a stool near my head. A patchwork of white and green clothing gathered closely around me. The staff physician, Dr. P., leaned toward me and said, "We're going to give you a Tensilon test in a minute, okay?" He picked up my left arm in his. "I want you to pull toward you as hard as you can. Okay. Good. Now we'll go ahead." He drew up a syringe, cleaned off a port on my IV line and injected a clear substance into the tube.

Within seconds, my stomach churned and my face striated with pain. My eyelids opened wide, but I lost focus. My eyeballs seemed to roll uncontrollably in my head. "Yeow!" I vocalized weakly.

He lifted up my arm: "Pull towards you." He nodded to everyone. "See that? And look at her heart rate—it's dropped." He looked at me emphatically. "That," he said, "is one of the more dramatic responses I've ever seen." His face quieted. "Young lady, you have myasthenia gravis. You're going to the T. W. hospital to get plasmapheresis." As the crowd dispersed, he paused and placed his hand on mine: "We know what you've got."

The head nurse bowed her blonde head toward mine in the bed. "I know you've had a rough time in the last few years. But the mystery's over. It's gonna be okay."

Dr. P. glanced at her, "You'll arrange the transfer?" He watched me for a second. "And call anesthesiology. She needs to be intubated again. She's working too hard." He looked at Aruna briefly, "Okay...that's it," and then turned away.

Myasthenia gravis. Ordinarily this would be nothing to rejoice over. But I did. Perhaps, I thought, as I lay mired in the flood of my paralysis, I need no longer be completely afraid. Maybe I could stop being hypervigilant and relax. Perhaps, I could begin to trust—to trust, just a little—that I might be cared for rather than rebuffed.

The next day, a bevy of attendants jostled me into the back of an ambulance. The vehicle wended its way through rush hour traffic. Occasionally, I saw the slow flash of lights reflected against the sides of trucks and streetcars as we passed.

T. W. hospital's ICU was large and dark. As I was transferred into a bed, I felt a pang of fear as unfamiliar faces advanced toward me. The head of the ICU walked over and introduced himself. "Hi, I'm Dr. Q.," he said. He picked up my hand and put it in his and added, "We don't mollycoddle patients like they do over at W. hospital." His brisk manner intimidated me. "I don't believe in keeping people here any longer than they should be," he said. He pulled back the bed sheet and began to examine me. After several minutes he looked at me, "Let's pull the NG tube. You don't need it.... Then maybe a bit later we'll see how you do without the vent. Maybe tomorrow we can stop the nitro as well."

With a nurse's assistance, he rolled my body on its side. "You're already getting skin breakdown," he said. Addressing the nurse, he directed, "She's to be turned every two hours, and for the first twenty-four hours only side to side, not on her back." He settled me back onto a pillow: "Oh yeah, I want physio and OT to see her.... Okay. That's it for the moment. The neuro team should be in to see you sometime." He reached for his clipboard that was resting at the end of the bed. "Let's see if we can get you upstairs in the next couple of days. I'll see you later."

The next morning, the vent was withdrawn, and by the afternoon I was extubated. Again, I could breathe but only shallowly and with immense effort. I still couldn't speak. A neurology resident came to see me. He stood at the end of my bed, reading through sheaves of paper and binders. He left without addressing me. Late in the evening, I was transferred upstairs to the neurology ward. As I left the ICU, a respiratory therapist reminded me, "Your volumes are low. Try to breathe more often and more deeply."

My new room was next to the nursing station. I could hear phones ringing and the thump of administrative machinery. Through the open doorway, I caught snatches of conversations. In the bed next to me, a young woman lay recovering from Guillain-Barré syndrome. Although she was still somewhat paralyzed from the waist down, her spirits were high. She had been on a ventilator a few weeks ago but now chatted sanguinely on the telephone by her bed. Her television flashed through the hanging cloth divider. Wafts of hospital and junk food permeated the room. Three or four members of her family and friends sat and visited.

The commotion felt barely tolerable. I lay mute and motionless, concentrating on inhaling and expelling air. I stared at the pastel-colored print of a clown that was screwed into the pale green wall. My throat ached sharply from the memory of the tubes. I grew afraid to sleep.

A nurse brushed back the curtain and gaped at me blankly. She was asthmatic—I could hear faint wheezing from where I was lying. She told me that she'd be back in a while to settle me for the night and then disappeared.

During the next twenty-four hours, I fought exhaustion. While I had begun to be able to turn my head, this mobility slowly ebbed. Saliva pooled in my throat, my jaw hung slackly, and my eyelids began to lower more. My chest seemed more rigid with each hour that passed. Cut off and alone, I resolved to try to keep breathing. And then gradually, I realized I was slipping. In the corridor, I could hear the mundane chorus of nursing chores and accompanying chatter. I tried to move my hand against the call bell and failed. I tried again and heard the bell ring in the distance. It was quickly shut off. I rolled my hand again against the sensor. The bell rang. I heard a voice say, "She probably wants to be moved. Can someone tell her I'll be in in a minute?" The bell shut off. I pressed once more. Finally, I heard squeaking footsteps penetrate my room.

"Oh God, hon!" I felt the nurse begin to raise the head of the bed. "It's okay. We're going to help you breathe. Hold on."

I felt an increased flow of oxygen hiss through the mask resting on my face.

"Hey, I need some help in here! I need the 'sat' monitor."

Within seconds a tumult of activity invaded my room. Fluorescent ceiling lights blazed through my lowered eyelids.

"Her 'sats' are low. Get ICU back up here."

Another voice called out, "Get me a suction kit—her airway needs clearing."

A hand rested on my forehead: "We may need to bag you, hon."

Within a few minutes, a woman resident arrived from ICU and readmitted me. "But," she cautioned, "you're going to have to stay here a couple of more hours until we can clear beds. In the meantime, Dr. R. from hematology is coming to see you—you're lucky, we got him just before he was leaving for dinner. He's going to arrange for plasmapheresis." As she left I heard her comment to someone, "Don't worry, I'm on the crash team if anything happens."

When Dr. R. arrived, I managed to lift my left eyelid just enough to glimpse his rumpled trousers and the bottom of his lab coat. He leaned over the bed and lifted my eyelids with his fingertips. He loomed blurrily over me. "We're going to put a shunt into your chest here," he indicated. "Then we're going to strain off your white blood cells and then remix your red cells with fresh plasma. It looks like egg white and comes from other people. There's a small risk of hepatitis and HIV infection. But the albumin is pasteurized, so it's unlikely." He paused. "Any questions?"

I tried turning my wrist.

"Can she talk?" He queried the nurse sitting next to me.

"No, but maybe she can write."

"Can she sign her name?" He put a marker in my hand. "Here, if you agree, sign right here on the bottom of this page."

With the pen, I slowly inked "CHOICE?" on the sheet.

"Are there any other choices? That's what you want to know? I don't think so. Plasmapheresis is it."

I signed my initials.

Within the next few minutes a resident inserted a large IV underneath my clavicle. He attached what felt like a large electrical plug to the shunt and sutured the whole thing to my chest. Soon I was back in intensive care being prepped to be reintubated. Dr. Q. again held my hand in his, "It's okay. We're just going to hook you back up to a ventilator."

Internally, I screamed with panic. I couldn't bear the thought of the tube again—if they could just help me breathe without lodging a hard plastic hose in my throat.[1] I flexed my wrist over and over trying to get his attention.

He placed a pen in my hand. I tried to write.

After a few seconds, he looked at the pad, "I can't read it. Try again."

I tried to write more legibly.

"I can't make it out." He deliberated. "Look, make a mark if you agree to be ventilated."

I didn't move.

"You mean, you don't want to be ventilated?"

I marked the paper.

"Oh..." I could feel him massage my hand a little in his. "What happens if you crash; will you let us resuscitate you?"

A mournful ache spread through me. If I was quite literally dying, I would endure the pain. I moved the pen.

"Let's be clear. You will let us resuscitate you?"

I moved the pen again.

"Okay. Good. Then I want to measure your neck for the tube and I am going to leave it right here—on the table beside you—in case we need it."

At one point, my nurse leaned down and said, "I've been reading the chart. You're not really sick. Dr. Q.'s overreacting. He should send you back upstairs." I heard her remark to a nurse at the neighboring bed, "She doesn't belong in ICU."

Great, the staff disagreed—how reassuring. I prayed for her shift to end.

Interspersed lines from a Theodore Roethke poem about a child clinging on to his drunken father reeled round and round my brain: "But I

---

1. This hospitalization took place in 1996. Now external breathing apparatuses (e.g., BiPAP and CPAP) are used in ICUs to assist with weak respiration. These do not require intubation.

hung on like death: / Such waltzing was not easy." An old friend came to see me. He looked exhausted, having flown in from Japan the same day. With the remaining strength in my hand, I hung on to him.

Plasmapheresis treatments began the next day. I felt an immediate change in my body. I understood that the distinction was imperceptible to the people around me, but I knew it. I felt it. The clamps that had seized down on every fiber of my body loosened very slightly. My saliva even tasted different.

Later that day I was transferred to a more chronic area of the unit. Through eavesdropping, I discovered that a comatose man lay to my left and, in the opposite corner, a young man lay encased by Guillain-Barré. Both of them were ventilated through tracheostomies.

My hearing was becoming extraordinarily acute. Very quickly I could not only tell the footfall of the various respiratory therapists, nurses, orderlies, and physicians, I could predict which room they would choose to enter from the subtle variations in the patterns of their treads. My sense of smell was also heightened. The aroma of various crushed medicines wafted toward me from across the room. With a new NG tube in place, I knew precisely which medications were being prepared for me as well as for the other patients. Scents and sounds allowed me to access and interpret much of my world, even as my eyelids were now almost completely sealed.

Unfortunately, I could also hear the arguments in the hallway between the physicians about my case. "Her toes curled up yesterday. They aren't today."

"Are you sure?"

"I dunno know. I think so....No, I'd swear it."

"She has a lot of clonus."

"Dr. S. won't do the evokeds again. She's negative. W. hospital probably just screwed up the Tensilon."

"I don't believe she has myasthenia."

"Well, someone does, cause she's on the meds."

"Who ordered the plasma anyway?"

"Dr. Q. did."

"What you bet she took something that we can't trace? They say she's really bright."

Aruna overheard a neurology resident discussing my case in the elevator that day. The tone of the discussion was one of mixed revulsion, anger, awe, and confusion.

Every few hours, Dr. Q. would stop by my bed. He would lift the covers and ask, "Can you move anything? Show me what you can do?"

After the second plasma course, my eyelids lifted slightly. But my pulmonary capacity remained marginal. I worked terribly hard to move small volumes of air. I still couldn't speak, swallow, or shut my mouth. Dr. Q. remarked, "You look exhausted. Too scared to sleep, eh?" He tried to reassure me, "You can sleep. If you stop breathing, we'll resuscitate you."

Weeks of struggle wore me down. I was no longer sure I could endure the tube in my throat.

The next plasma round improved me more markedly. Dr. Q. commented that I had more expression in my face. An odd pain began to invade my body. I managed to write this to him.

"I know you probably won't like to hear this, but increased pain is a good sign." He smiled. "It really is."

Dr. Q. seemed to intuit my concerns. "I've got an idea. Your eyes seem better. You can focus a bit?" He paused. "Okay. My orders are for the nursing station TV and VCR to be brought in. I'm going to get your nurse here to call your family to bring in as many movies as they can find."

His suggestion buoyed me.

"It's completely understandable that this is getting to you. You've been here a long time." His hand rested on my ankle. "And I'm going to call the pain management team.... We're looking at longer-term pain control. They're better at that than I am."

A few days later, as I awaited more plasmapheresis, Dr. Q. came to say good-bye. "I've been here for longer than my usual stint," he said. Dr. T. is taking over for the next couple of weeks. After that I'll be back. But, I think you may be upstairs by then. He'll take good care of you." In his usual manner, he held my hand in his. "Before I go, is there anything you need or want?" He bent his ear to my mouth.

"How long will I be like this?" I managed to whisper.

"Honestly? I don't know. I really don't know."

Two days later, I was transferred back to neurology. My breathing seemed more stable. I could vocalize weakly. My left arm was a bit more mobile and I could turn my head to one side. I still required a feeding tube, which, if it was run too quickly, backed liquid feedings out through my nose and mouth. I couldn't roll myself over or sit up.

Now that I was on the neurology ward, I had little contact with the physicians who were overseeing my care. I knew that they were reluctant to have me there.

They left orders for me to be sat up in an elongated "geri" chair for fifteen to twenty minutes a day. The chair itself was large, with armrests, and could be reclined quite far back. Because I had so few active muscles, I had to be tied into it. Even my head was secured by straps across my forehead and chin. While I had been subjected to this type of exercise in ICU, a respiratory therapist and nurse were always present to ensure I didn't pass out or stop breathing. On the ward, two nurses transferred and tied me into the chair. Before they departed, they left an oxygen mask on my face and a call bell next to the hand I couldn't move. But, because I still couldn't speak, I mutely endured this error.

Being in the reclined chair totally exhausted me. Perspiration drenched my gown. After a while, I felt terrible. I hoped someone would come back. I could hear footsteps intermittently in the hall. No one came. I started to retch and what little focus I had disappeared. My breathing was terribly shallow and slow. The straps holding me up dug into me with increasing sharpness as my body slumped against them. I knew that I was on the verge of unconsciousness—an unconsciousness that would kill me because I would stop breathing. I focused every aspect of my will and being on remaining conscious—on inhaling and on exhaling. I retched again . . . and again. I tried to telepathically urge one of the passing footsteps in the corridor to turn in at my door. Finally, a nurse returned. She looked at my ashen, sweating visage and commented nonchalantly, "You look a little tired." She fiddled with the covers on my bed. "I have to wait 'til Joanie comes to help me put you back to bed."

If I could have wept and begged her to hurry, I would have. Instead, I implored myself to hang on.

She stood beside me and placed a hand on my shoulder, "Ooo, your gown is soaking! You're sweating a lot." She paused, "You know I have that problem too. I even use a special cream from my doctor…though I think I'm going to try acupuncture. I hear it works." Her hand brushed my neck, "I'll get you a clean gown once we put you in bed."

At last, Joanie trotted into the room, her shoes squeaking slightly against the tile floor.

I continued to urge myself to hold on.

Finally, they undid me and half-lifted and half-dragged me into the bed. Joanie commented, "Whew, you don't look so good—that tired you out I bet!" She rubbed my forearms and face, "Those straps have left red marks in your skin. Maybe we should get an ice pack so they don't leave a bruise."

After replacing my hospital gown, they tucked an array of pillows in around me and then left.

Being on the bed was a relief. But, while I felt a little more stable, I still felt precarious. Very gradually the sense that I was about to founder dissipated. About half an hour later, Joanie returned. "Well, you look a lot better now," she said. Maybe tomorrow they shouldn't leave you up so long."

Dr. S., the neurologist who had visited me a couple of times in intensive care, stopped in very early one morning. Aruna stood by my bed, sharing the news from home before heading off to work. He shut the door to my room. "Look," he said, "I believe you have myasthenia, but most of my colleagues don't. You have a long and complex medical history." He paced back and forth at the end of my bed. "Over the years, practically every neurologist has had contact with your case. I can't treat you for myasthenia if I don't have the support of my colleagues. The one physician who sees myasthenics has refused you as a patient." He looked stern. "I'm sorry, but there's very little I can do in these circumstances. The plasma exchanges will go on for only a couple of more times. I won't be able to reorder them."

I couldn't believe this, yet I had no way to argue against it as my eyes brimmed with tears.

"I'm sorry." He stepped toward the door. "And, if you ever say we had this conversation, I will deny it." He opened it and left.

A clinical detachment characterized my stay on the ward. During morning rounds little was said about my condition. Occasionally, I would be asked by some doctor whether I thought I was ready to go home yet. He or she would remind me that my hospital stay had been long and expensive. I felt like shooting them all and began to dread the arrival of any doctor by my bedside.

In the meantime, I continued with physiotherapy and occupational therapy. Over a period of three months, I began to have more movement. My speaking voice started to return. Finally, after several swallowing studies, it was determined that my feeding tube could be withdrawn. Every so often, when I pushed too hard, the paralysis would slip back and I would have a bit more difficulty. Nonetheless, I was making steady progress.

At the beginning of the fourth month, two residents approached me about being transferred to a rehabilitation hospital. I agreed and signed a consent form. Within the week, a nurse, a physiotherapist, and Dr. M. from the spinal cord rehab hospital came to assess me. I knew and liked all of them. I knew that they also liked me. Dr. M. summarized their position: "We know you will work hard. We've seen it before. But you're still pretty weak. And, as you know, we don't deal with patients who need to be ventilated."

"But, I haven't been intubated in weeks," I protested.

"Yes, I know. But you're breathing still doesn't look that secure. You tire very easily." She cradled a binder in her arms. "We *will* take you," she emphasized. "But, in a few more weeks, when you're stronger. Be patient."

The following day, a social worker came in to tell me, "Since you are a poor rehab candidate, I'm here to arrange transfer to a nursing home."

"But I want to go to rehab. I don't want to go into a nursing home."

"Well, the rehab hospital didn't take you. Anyway, you signed the consent form."

"I did not!"

"It's on the same form as the request for rehab placement."

"But the chronic care stuff was separate. I didn't check it off."

"Well, there's a check mark beside it now." She seemed frustrated and confused. "It will probably take a few weeks for a bed to come up, so it won't happen immediately. Maybe you should talk to your doctor if you don't want to go."

I complained to the female resident who saw me the next morning.

She seemed irritated, "You've been here a long time. You're blocking a bed. We tried to get you into rehab, as you requested. But they won't take you." She persisted, "You've got yourself into quite a situation. But we can't keep you here. You are not a medical case. There are people who are really and truly sick, who need this bed."

Two days later my nurse didn't come in with my scheduled medication. I asked for my pills. She informed me that most of my meds were being discontinued. The aim was to have me weaned from all medication within two weeks.

Slowly, I was gaining new capacities. I could roll myself in bed. With the help of a long, angled spoon, I could feed myself the mashed potatoes and minced beef that seemed to constitute my hospital diet. I didn't want to get worse. Yet, even as I felt more fearful that I would be paralyzed again, I tried to calm myself. Perhaps, I thought, it would be wise to see whether the medications really helped. I counseled myself to be patiently watchful—to wait and see what happened. Moreover, I knew that I couldn't expect my physicians to prescribe drugs that they themselves were unsure of.

Within a couple of days the reduced dosages started to take a toll. To both nurses and therapists my body seemed heavier. I found it more difficult to move and focus my eyes. My eyelids began to descend. I tired more easily. A few days later, all chemical therapies were stopped and I felt my body sag more heavily. By the end of the following week, I found it difficult to speak and swallow. One day, shortly after physiotherapy, I struggled to breathe and grew frightened. An ICU resident came to see me and offered to move me back downstairs for the night. I feared the pain of an intubation and refused.

The following morning, with my face and body increasingly paralyzed, I asked to see my attending physician. The female resident arrived instead. She stood at the end of my bed.

"I don't think I can take this experiment for much longer," I said. "I would like you to restart my medications."

"Why?"

"I'm getting weaker."

"I don't see it."

"Well, my physio and OT see it. The nurses do, too."

"We are not giving you any medications. You're not sick." She rapped a knuckle against her clipboard. "And doctors *prescribe*, nurses do *not*. You may be able to convince others, but you will not convince us!"

"Can't you see my face? My eyelids are almost closed. I have trouble seeing clearly."

"I don't believe you." She paused and then spoke again. "Most myasthenics can move their eyebrows even when the rest of their face is paralyzed. Let's see you do that." She waited.

I tried to wriggle my eyebrows but they remained stiffly glued in place.

"You see, you didn't move them."

"I can't move them!"

"No. It's just that you don't want to move them! And you say that your eyesight is blurred, but it's not."

"It is."

"No, it isn't."

The futility of my plea cascaded within me. "So you won't re-prescribe the drugs?"

"No."

I felt close to tears. A protective emotional shell began to descend about me. "I guess there's nothing more to say."

"No. We're arranging for transfer to a nursing facility as soon as possible."

We stared at each other in a piqued silence. She turned and left the room.

During the afternoon, Aruna and I decided to take me home. With the help of insurance, we booked private nursing care. The following morning I informed the physicians who made rounds. They seemed concurrently irked and relieved. "We do not think that this is in your best interest. Perhaps, your partner is poisoning you and that is why you are sick....Maybe she has Munchausen syndrome by proxy."

This was something new, and I couldn't believe it. I would have scoffed at the stupidity of their suggestion if it hadn't had such dangerous implications.[2] Although I understood that Aruna's commitment to me stigmatized her to some degree, the doctors were on the verge of criminalizing her. I knew I had to quash this suggestion as quickly and as firmly as possible. I angrily responded by reminding them: "If you look at the chart you will realize that my paralysis and weakness started years before we met."

"Are you sure? Are you sure she isn't poisoning you? It could be detrimental to your health for you to go home," they cautioned.

My resolve hardened against them. "No," I simply replied. But it was becoming clear to me that it was actually becoming dangerous for me—and for Aruna—to remain under their "care."

Up until this point, I was thought to have a psychosomatic disorder, an unconscious manifestation of physical symptoms. My years as a "not yet diagnosed" patient had taught me that despite the distinction between unconscious and willed disorders, physicians tended to conflate the two and treat psychosomatic patients as though they were willfully responsible for their symptoms. Now they were accusing Aruna of trying to kill me.

---

2. Munchausen syndrome is a psychiatric disorder in which symptoms are consciously produced by patients to gain some form of internal gratification or attention from others. Munchausen's by proxy (MSP) is an extension of this disorder as it applies to caregivers who deliberately exaggerate, fabricate, and/or induce health problems in others to gain some form of internal gratification or attention from others for their caregiving.

14 Contemplating Hemlock

Within two days, I lay in my own bed. While my family physician agreed to restart medications for myasthenia gravis, I was still very ill, and Aruna and I were utterly alone. We knew that the general proviso was that somatizing patients should not have access to more than the bare minimum of medical care because access to medical resources would only legitimate the erroneous belief that they were ill. Given the sheer depth and degree of my incapacity during the past weeks, along with the positive Tensilon test administered in the ICU, we thought that this might have finally redirected the ethos and trajectory of my medical care—but it hadn't. It was readily apparent that even when I was dying or severely incapacitated, we could not confidently turn to the health-care system for assistance. The stigma of a psychosomatic diagnosis was so powerful that it overwhelmed even concrete evidence of my failing vital signs. Moreover, when we later asked for copies of the charts from Montreal and this latest hospitalization, the emergency room notes and a portion of the ICU notes for both charts had been lost and were labeled as "missing."[1] This seemed highly coincidental to both ourselves and my GP.

1. These pages were still missing even two to three years later when we reissued our requests. My hospital charts from Toronto also had "lost" sections.

What was perhaps most galling was the confirmation of our suspicion that the poor care I received was not just the result of my having bizarre symptoms but was also the product of political disputes and territoriality between physicians. The fact that diagnostic errors had occurred early on and had then been replicated over and over with the centralization of medical resources meant that it was now too difficult for a physician who wished to remedy the error to go against the accrued weight of medical opinion. The classification that I finally seemed to fit into—albeit atypically—was a neurological one, but the neurology community firmly disavowed me and it. For example, I had only received plasmapheresis at the behest of doctors in the ICU and not because it was ordered by neurologists. In short, the system was too invested in its understanding of me as psychologically unbalanced and thus was unable to reconstruct that view or revise its plan.

Deeply disillusioned and fearful that I might well lapse into another crisis to which I would once again receive an embattled and ambivalent response, Aruna and I began to explore death and dying societies. I had spent the previous eighteen months largely bedridden, aching with pain, fatigue, and paralysis. I was so infirm that I sprained my joints when I tried to lift or roll myself. Often, I was too weak to eat or speak. My endurance was waning. The image of a quick death comforted me, but I worried about becoming too weak to kill myself.

We contacted two different organizations that counseled people with chronic or fatal illnesses about techniques for euthanasia. Typically, we were told, individuals stockpiled narcotics and/or muscle relaxants and then took an overdose. The individual would also place a plastic bag over his or her head and seal it around the neck with an elastic band. There were vague suggestions that a trusted companion might have to hold the bag down when the patient reflexively reached to free his or herself. Confronted by the messy reality of such a venture, the prospect of killing me became an enormous psychological and physical challenge. In no way did we want Aruna to struggle with plastic bags or pillows in order to smother me. Moreover, given my uncertain stomach, it was likely that my system wouldn't absorb the narcotics before it finally ejected them. Consequently, one counselor suggested that we find a vet who might be willing to provide intramuscular (i.e., injectable) medicines and thus make the whole process less violent and the outcome more certain. In the end, our exploration of the details of euthanasia did little to comfort us. It was theoretically attractive, but an immersion in the concrete details discouraged us.

We agreed to wait a couple of weeks to see whether I gained any strength from the resumption of my drugs. And, in fourteen days, I did make gains.

Unfortunately, during the third week, I ate strawberries that were infested with cyclospora. I became terribly weak and ill. On television, the evening news reported the local outbreak. Even as I became more and more dehydrated and struggled to breathe, we knew we would not call a doctor or ambulance. The private duty nurse called her supervisor and whispered anxiously that I was dying. It was not until many months later that my partner confessed her fear that she would either come home to or wake up to a cold corpse during this period.

Fortunately, I survived the food poisoning. And during the next months I continued to improve. The combination of pyridostigmine and corticosteroids nourished me. I gained movement, muscle mass, and physical energy. My GP became more aggressive in treating me and added another drug to my regimen in order to strengthen my immune suppression. During the next four months, I went from using a power chair to a manual one. And then, within another three months I stood, teetering, on my legs. Soon, I was taking pained steps. It was the first time I had walked in four to five years. My progress was uneven but steady. I had days that set me back. I tired easily, and my joints and muscles often hurt from the new efforts. But internally, I clutched tenaciously to the prospect of a return to healthy functioning. And I improved.

One evening I was out in my manual wheelchair with my children. As we turned into a bike shop, a hand tapped me on the shoulder. I turned around and before me stood one of the residents from the intensive care unit. He couldn't disguise the astonishment on his face. "I've been following you for a couple of blocks. You…you…look amazing," he stuttered. "I can't believe it!"

"I know. I feel pretty good."

We chatted a bit more, and then he finally exclaimed, "God, now I know we make a difference! I really thought you would die." We shook hands. I thanked him. He walked away, his face lit up by an enormous grin.

15 *Icarus*

My recovery was a rebirth. I had been in a crucible of suffering for many years. I emerged from this with a chronic and gnawing fear of dying—not of death, but of dying. I had lain, expiring, for weeks in ICU, and I did not think I could bear to take that on again. The only downside to being alive, I reasoned, was that it meant that I must at some point die. Death was not the problem—dying, however, was. Dying was lonely and painful. So, even as I got better, I was shadowed by this silent morbid anxiety. All I could hope was that my apprehension would disappear as I encountered increased and sustained health.

At the same time I was also consumed by another overawing force: an enormous sexual appetite engulfed me. In the past, Aruna's passion and capacity for sex had almost always outstripped mine. Now, however, I wanted to have sex four or five times a day—sometimes even more. There was no way that my spouse could keep pace with the urgency and frequency of my new arousal. It was as if my body understood that it had just barely survived—that it had lived for months, even years, on a knife-edge of existence—and now it was determined to reproduce itself before it died. This was the only rational explanation I could think of. The ecstatic impulse lasted several months and then gradually settled down.

Thanks to being properly medicated with immune suppressants and drugs to facilitate nerve-muscle junctions, after about six months, I began to walk with some consistency and distance. In all the years we had been together, Aruna, Justin, and Alisha had never seen me walk—this was an extraordinarily poignant time for us as a family. We decided to move out of our accessible flat as it was very expensive—our rent consumed two-thirds of our monthly income. As well, now our activities were no longer circumscribed by whether we could negotiate wheelchair access. Admittedly, some days were better than others. I often had pain and fatigue, which meant I had to use a manual wheelchair or crutches. But as long as I rested often and took my medications, we could all revel in the mundane aspects of everyday life. I even began to teach the children to ski the following winter. (This has since become a beloved family activity.)

Crucially, I finally had the physical stamina to renew work on my doctoral dissertation. The scholarly realm had sustained me during times of enormous pain and struggle, and I approached my PhD with a re-animated vigor. But both the trauma and drama of the previous years blocked me psychologically. I did not know how I would write a highly theorized and critical account of power in medical practice given my marginal status as a patient. It seemed impossible for me to write on the topic without somehow revealing the nature of my own illness and contact with the medical profession. But I found it very difficult, if not impossible, to speak of my so-called somatic tendencies to anyone but Aruna. Even though I no longer believed that I had a conversion disorder, its presence in my medical chart could still evoke a sense that I was somehow fraudulent and delusional—and, these feelings kept me from moving forward in my writing.

My journey as a patient had not only been about my symptoms but it had also been about the conflicted mooting of what was wrong with me. I loathed the psychosomatic diagnosis—but it was central to my medical care. Moreover, it had very nearly killed me. Though in the past both Aruna and I had used Medline—an electronic medical database—to pull up articles on conversion and dissociative disorders, we had never really read through the materials in a sustained or methodical manner—at the time, the content often angered or alienated us. I soon realized that I would have to turn and face my enemy. I knew that I could not be an effective critic of medicine without disclosing the fact that many doctors did not view me as legitimately ill.

So, even though I felt a gross discomfort with the topic, I metaphorically held my breath and leapt into reading medical articles. After perusing periodicals from the latter part of the twentieth century, I reached back into the history of the illness. I read Sigmund Freud's collected works, concentrating particularly on his two seminal cases of conversion disorder (i.e., hysteria): Anna O. and Dora. That these two inconclusive cases formed the basis of the current medical understanding of psychosomatic illness stunned me. I struggled through the nineteenth-century French texts of Martin Charcot and others. I even dredged up some medieval sources on witches, whom some feminist critics believe to be some of the early hysterics or somatizers. I then worked forward chronologically, revisiting more contemporary books and articles.

I found myself contesting even feminist scholars' understanding of psychogenic illness. Elaine Showalter, a renowned feminist critic, argues that the female hysterics of the nineteenth century unconsciously rebelled against the rigid strictures of Victorian society. They became ill and took to their beds as a way to bypass the patriarchal duties being thrust on them. But I found this interpretation actually confirmed the medical presumption that these women were difficult and antisocial. From my perspective, Showalter validates the misogynist views of physicians when confronted by "functional" illnesses. The feminist therapist Judith Herman points to psychosomatic illnesses, such as post-traumatic stress disorder (among others), as a way of privileging subjective narrative in the clinic. But I couldn't support this view, for over the years, I found that my own subjective narrative had been constantly called up and then dissected by the objectifying gaze of medical staff. In the end, most of what I encountered only helped to reinforce the painful observations and criticisms I arrived at as a patient—the various sources served to support my growing skepticism about the efficacy of current approaches to (and treatments of) somatoform disorders.

From 1960 until the present, an ambivalence emerges in the medical literature between those who believe that these disorders exist and those who believe they don't. Ironically, my own position comes down simultaneously on both sides. Illness is a whole experience, and so it truly encompasses all of the body, mind, emotions, and spirit. In an effort to make illness more manageable in our daily lives we tend to parcel it off as "just a cold" or a "sprained ankle." But even these innocuous ailments affect us more than just physically. For example, I've experienced psychological side effects from antinausea medications that have made me intolerably agitated. Furthermore, I know that pain thins my concentration and makes me irritable. Likewise, when I am weak or I have involuntary muscles twitches that last for days, depression stalks me and reduces my capacity to endure these symptoms. But despite these confirmations of psyche-soma links, I do *not* believe that the psyche is capable of creating dire and prolonged physical illness. Furthermore, I believe that the diagnostic category of somatoform disorders is largely a cultural artifact masquerading as a medical truth.

I will try to explain this a bit more clearly: In the past five years I confronted a similar cultural bias masquerading as psychological truth when my youngest two children were born. I had presumed that as infants they would occupy a nearby bassinet in our bedroom and that they would then move to their own crib and bed in an adjacent room. I fully believed that I would let my children "cry it out" and that they would then be capable of "self-soothing" themselves to sleep. But once my children were born, my assumptions crumbled in the face of their vulnerability. It seemed impractical to have them sleep anywhere but with us—easier for them to nurse and much easier on our sleep schedules! Moreover, I realized that I knew of no species of animal that slept apart from its offspring. I also finally noticed that the vast majority of people in the world sleep with their children. Given that our wealthy, modern, and liberal society can afford multiple bedrooms, we can chose to bed our children separately, but we are the anomaly. My youngest child was less than six months old when the devastating tsunami of 2004 struck the Indian Ocean, and I knew that if a similar disaster struck our own family, I would want my children within arm's reach and not in an adjacent room (even if I could not save them). I also noticed that much of the parenting and medical literature echoed the discourse of liberal doctrine, speaking of the need to create "psychologically healthy and independent" children. This emphasis on independence, freedom, and autonomy comes directly from liberal philosophers such as John Locke, John Stuart Mill, and John Rawls. The paradigm of self-possessed, self-controlled, and autonomous individuals pervades our society and infiltrates medical and scientific literature, where it is treated as a norm or as fact. It is a metanarrative in which we all take part but barely notice.

As I've outlined previously, the psychologizing of disease dovetails with these liberal models. When popular and medical culture speaks of "holistic" approaches to illness and disease, it usually means that these approaches embody an alternate attitude toward human illness. As patients, by acknowledging our feelings, it is assumed that we can become more self-aware and thereby encourage our own healing. But a closer examination reveals that the belief that one can improve oneself psychologically, and thus physically, actually parallels a mainstream discourse that champions individual liberty and mastery. But instead of being free and autonomous consumers, producers, and voters who actively construct and control the world we live in, patients are presented as self-conscious beings who, by seeking and gaining emotional control and enlightenment, defeat whatever ails them (whether it is cancer, heart disease, or inexplicable paralysis). As such, psychological theories of disease do not provide alternate discourses and paradigms; they are, rather, firmly embedded in the mainstream of liberal, technocratic Western and medical culture.

Moreover, as medicine tries to transform itself to be more responsive to patients' needs, it uses psychological theories to bolster its efforts to combat illness and disease. But I wonder about these well-intentioned efforts. It seems to me that, despite the new rhetoric, the Cartesian divide between mind and body remains rigidly in place in hospitals. (Susan Sontag, a social critic and a highly experienced cancer patient, also found these trends to be misguided.) If an ailment is organic (or "real"), it is treated by physical medicine specialists. But if an ailment is functional, it immediately becomes the sole purview of the psychiatrists. Being human and being sick means the whole being is involved, but the divide between psychiatry and the rest of the hospital remains constant. So if you are schizophrenic and happen to get ovarian cancer, the likelihood is that your oncologists will feel very uncomfortable dealing with you as a patient because they know little or nothing about "diseases of the mind." Moreover, your cancer may well not be detected and treated immediately because it will initially be presumed that your symptoms are psychiatric. The stigma of mental and emotional illness remains strong in medicine. Most poignant, even though neurologists and psychiatrists both deal with diseases of the mind/brain, the divide between the two fields remains strong. The separation between the two was traditionally an organic-functional one. But as some mental illnesses (i.e., bipolar disorder and schizophrenia) are increasingly shown to be chemical (and maybe genetic) malfunctions of the brain (in other words, they have physical, "real" causes), they nonetheless remain within psychiatry—I suspect that this is due to both historical convention and the inappropriate social behaviors associated with these disorders. In sum, there may be new psychological discourses about illness, but the actual arrangement of specialties means that physicians are really ill-equipped to respond to patients in a truly holistic manner.

Interestingly, as I read my way through various medical journal articles on psychosomatic illness, I discovered that a noticeable percentage of them were written by Canadians or by physicians in Canadian hospitals. All of these authors seemed to believe that somatoform disorders exist and that the best treatments are ones in which the patient is "discouraged" from adopting a sick role. Moreover, two physicians based in London, Ontario, Robert Teasell and Allan Shapiro, run a clinic that treats psychogenic illnesses. In 2004, they not only argued that behavioral modification is the best method with which to treat these disorders but also they advocated placing patients in a double bind. The treating medical team (composed of therapists, nurses, social workers, and doctors) tells the patient that if symptoms subside and disappear then his or her illness is organic (and thereby legitimate), but if the symptoms persist, then his or her illness must be functional (and thus not legitimate) (Teasel and Shapiro, 2004). Additionally, patients who stubbornly remain ill have privileges such as television and telephone withdrawn and contact with family and friends prohibited. Those that recover gain these "freedoms." Unfortunately, Teasell and Shapiro have had difficulty tracking the long-term outcomes of patients of their clinic. Patients seem (understandably) to disappear or refuse to respond to queries after they have been discharged. So it is largely unknown whether the "cures" achieved in the short term sustain themselves in the long term.

Interestingly, it is quite well known that individuals initially diagnosed with conversion reactions are found to have an organic disease at a later date. During the 1950s and 1960s this incidence ran as high as 20 percent of cases. More recently, it is believed that "misdiagnosis" of conversion reaction has fallen to between 4 and 7 percent. But this still remains unacceptably high, especially when the authors note that one-third of these "psychosomatic" patients, when an attempt is made to contact them for follow-up, are discovered to have committed suicide (Stone et al., 2005). As such, Teasell and Shapiro's unit in London, Ontario, seems especially callous to me, for it does not allow any margin for those people who may well have a disease process that has evaded constructive diagnosis.

Having read these and other articles and having been unable to find a neurologist who would agree to follow me in Toronto or southern Ontario, I began to seriously wonder whether I might be better treated if I went to the United States. Perhaps a more staid Canadian medical and social culture lent itself to viewing my ailments as illegitimate. At different moments during the previous decade I had certainly fantasized about being able to take myself off to the Mayo Clinic in Rochester, Minnesota, or to some hotshot specialist at Harvard. But I had never had the physical and financial resources to do so.

But now Aruna and I decided it might be worth trying to confirm a diagnosis of myasthenia gravis at a notable American clinic. My current psychiatrist also thought that this might help me secure proper medical treatment in Toronto should I have another life-threatening crisis. He inquired about various neurologists and then arranged an appointment with a myasthenia expert on the East Coast.

Seated in a waiting room that harkened back to the modernism of the 1950s, I held all sorts of hope that this consultation would help me achieve some medical legitimacy and thus safeguard me during a crisis in the future. The myasthenia support group newsletter had described the physician, Dr. V., in glowing terms, and his patients seemed to regard him in an avuncular or grandfatherly manner.

It turned out that Dr. V. was a talkative man in his early sixties. During my initial examination, he administered a Tensilon test that he immediately and enthusiastically confirmed was positive. Ironically, the drug made me suddenly and profoundly weak so that I sank backward and couldn't speak. After a few moments, my strength returned. Dr. V. told me that this was a myasthenic response to an "overdose" of Tensilon— but it was a reaction I had never experienced! Dr. V. then assured me that all would now be well and that I should seriously contemplate having my thymus removed (a common, though little understood, treatment for myasthenics). He proposed that I undergo single-fiber EMG tests at a local hospital the following day.

I didn't want to spend limited funds on an unnecessary test and reminded him that I had never had a positive result. After much discussion, Dr. V. convinced me that others had not administered the test properly and that he had no doubt that I had myasthenia gravis but that he would need a single-fiber EMG to confirm his diagnosis. He would then make all the necessary arrangements for my future treatment. By the end of the afternoon I felt as though I was about to become a member of his extended family of myasthenic patients. He even began introducing me to other people in the waiting room and showed me the thymectomy scars at the base of their throats.

But the test the following day did not prove to be positive. When I met Dr. V. an hour or so later, his whole demeanor had changed. He acted as though I had carried out an elaborate scam. He did not like to think that he had been taken advantage of. He warned me that I needed serious psychiatric help, as it was impossible, in his view, for someone to have myasthenia gravis and not test positive on a single-fiber EMG. His antipathy was palpable. As I stood in his waiting room, counting out $1,200 in payment for his services to his nurse (it was equivalent at the time to about $1,500 in Canadian currency), I censored my desire to withhold his payment. I felt as though he had not properly listened to me. And now I had to pay him as he berated me. Out in the street, the city looked magnificent in the spring sunshine, but its marvels could not soothe my devastation. The crushing of my expectations rendered me mute. It took several hours before I could telephone Aruna with the bad news.

16 *A Crisis, American Style*

I returned to the nonspecialized care of my GP in Toronto. Within a year and half, I wrote and defended my doctoral dissertation. Our family now lived in a small semidetached house on a street near midtown. I still had fluctuations of strength and pain that were sometimes difficult to weather. But for the most part, my family and I were blissfully happy.

I now started to probe the academic job market. Much to my surprise, I won a Fulbright fellowship to study law in the United States. But for several weeks it seemed that I might not be able to take the esteemed fellowship because I couldn't qualify for the health insurance that the U.S. Immigration and Naturalization Service required of any visiting scholar. Fortunately, after a little research, we discovered that I was insured under Aruna's workplace plan, and so I successfully applied for an alien visa for academic travel and extended stay in the United States.

And so, in the fall of 1999, I rented the first floor of a house in Ithaca, New York, and began my postdoctoral studies at Cornell Law School. I commuted regularly back to Toronto to visit Aruna, Justin, and Alisha. We discovered that we didn't enjoy being apart and, consequently, we did our best to spend time as a family in either Ithaca or in Toronto. The academic year turned out to be one of my most memorable. My supervisor was one of the most generous colleagues and academics that I had ever encountered—a truly remarkable woman. I learned more and met more interesting people in one year than I had in the previous ten. It was a heartening experience.

But, in early April 2000, just as the spring was ripening into summer, my health began to falter. The day after I attended a three-day conference, at which I had presented a paper and spent hours listening to and commenting on other papers as well as dining out with colleagues, I retreated to my apartment in Ithaca feeling tired and unwell. In pain, I was soon very nauseated and vomiting. By midnight, I realized that I was dehydrated and losing movement and that, if I didn't act soon, I would be unable to call for help. I telephoned a friend and she drove me to the local hospital. The emergency room staff reacted swiftly—their concern was palpable. Once again I explained my ambiguous diagnosis: that I apparently suffered from a psychosomatic illness, which nevertheless responded well to treatments and protocols for myasthenia gravis.

Soon I was admitted to the "step down area" of the intensive care unit, which was also the edge of the pediatric ward. I hoped that this crisis would quickly pass, and so I hesitated to call Aruna and the children. I did not want to burden them unnecessarily when I was a four-to-five-hour's drive away. The attending neurologist examined me and told me that he believed I had MG. When my weakness intensified over the next day or so, he ordered IVIG (intravenous immunoglobulin). This is a blood product—human plasma—administered by IV, which is thought to calm overactive immune systems. It helped, but it did not shoot me back to my normal functioning. It now seemed best to telephone Aruna.

I stayed in the Ithaca hospital for several weeks. Dr. W., the physician who oversaw my care, visited me daily. In turn, my insurance company phoned *him* daily to inquire when I could be discharged or transferred back to a hospital in Ontario, Canada. Dr. W. felt trapped. He and the neurologist believed the one or two ten-day rounds of plasmapheresis was the best treatment. However, the relatively small hospital did not have the requisite equipment or staff to administer it. He wanted to transfer me to a larger hospital, but my insurance company refused to pay for the transfer. Its position was that if I was well enough to move, then I was well enough to be transferred back home (where they would no longer be responsible for financing my care). Consequently, Dr. W. spoke to neurologists in Toronto to find an open neurological bed. But no one was willing to take me. He was also reluctant to send me by ambulance to an ER in Toronto when my breathing could easily fail in transit. Moreover, he knew that it was unlikely that I would be treated as though I had myasthenia gravis. He argued intensively for days with the insurance company to allow a transfer within New York State. One morning he told me that if I deteriorated and needed ventilation, that is, life support, the insurance company would agree to such a move. But then he warned me with a shake of his forefinger that he would know I was really a "head case" if I deteriorated in the next day or so!

In the end, Dr. W. arranged for what he thought was a compassionate admission to a large teaching hospital in upstate New York. Apparently, a neurologist there was willing to treat me free of charge. The necessary plasmapheresis, it seemed, would be in place by the end of the week. Almost ecstatic, I called Aruna in Toronto. She promised to drive down to meet my ambulance at the hospital the following afternoon.

Because my respiratory capacity was unreliable, two paramedics accompanied me. The ambulance undulated up and down and swung from side to side as it navigated back roads. In the evening of an early June day, we finally pulled into what seemed a factorylike edifice. (I could see little from my stretcher.) Fortunately, Aruna had arrived about an hour earlier and had already been up to the neurology unit and seen the room to which I was to be admitted. She led the way through a maze of hallways and elevators.

When, at last, having turned a corner and waded through a series of doors, I caught sight of the ward, I was incredulous at what I saw: the neurology unit was almost a replica of a prison plan designed by Jeremy Bentham two centuries ago called "the Panopticon." In his plan there is a central tower surrounded by an outer ring of cells that are backlit by windows. Consequently, the warder can view the inmates from the central tower with total ease and the inmates are perennially visible to the jailer. Foucault references it in *Discipline and Punish* as an example of a type of invidious observation and total deprivation of privacy that can be imposed on individuals. The neurology ward was similar in that it had a central nursing station surrounded by rooms that had glass walls on their interior sides, facing the station. They also then had large windows that looked out onto the buildings and roofs of the rest of the hospital. This meant that the patients were constantly backlit and in profile to anyone at the circular nursing station. But, unfortunately, the layout did not make allowances for storage, and so the views from the nursing station were, in fact, obstructed by stretchers, IV poles, shelves of laundry, monitors, carts, wheelchairs, and a host of other medical equipment. The overall effect was one of chaotic messiness and inefficiency.

Immediately, I grasped that I had entered a behemoth of a hospital in which I would feel insignificant. I yearned for the close familiarity of the community hospital from which I had just been discharged. My worries grew as it took more than three hours before a nurse approached my bedside to formally admit me. If Aruna had not hovered nearby, I would not have had access to water or to the bathroom or even to be able to move myself on the bed.

Later in the evening, an admitting clerk arrived with forms for me to sign, which stated that I took full financial responsibility for all costs associated with my admission and care! When I inquired about my status as a "compassionate admission," no one seemed to know about it. The clerk reiterated that I must sign the papers. I refused. A pair of young residents came in to speak to me, they encouraged me to sign the forms and told me that I would not be able to receive any diagnostic tests or treatment unless I did so. Both the man and woman seemed uncomfortable, and I assumed that their awkwardness was due to a dislike of dealing with financial matters. Aruna and I consulted briefly, and once I had crossed out the paragraphs outlining my financial responsibilities, I finally initialed the sheet.

During the first hours, nurses gave me my myasthenia medications, but when I complained of pain, I received nothing. At the previous hospital, I had been on 90 milligrams of long-acting morphine twice a day, and I could ask for either oral or intramuscular short-acting morphine every few hours, if I became too uncomfortable. I was now in pain; moreover, my body was habituated to this dose. Without any morphine in my system, I began to have symptoms of withdrawal. My body felt weak, I sweated profusely, my eyes and nose ran, my muscles began to ache and twitch, I couldn't settle or sleep, and my pain began to resurge. I asked three or four times for pain relief, but the only clinical response was to increase the taking of my vital signs because my "blood pressure was acting up."

Just before Aruna left to check into a motel, the same two young physicians returned to my bedside with wry smirks and to say that they had received my chart from Toronto yesterday and that they knew "all about your illness," that they were "committed to providing me with the best care."

Aruna and I instantly understood that I might not only have to endure unsympathetic treatment but have to pay for it out of our own meager resources! Returning to Canada now seemed to be the best option. Until this moment, we both believed that, despite being far from home, my crisis was being better managed than it had been previously. We had thus not been too worried by the fact that my physicians had not been able to find a bed for me in Toronto. But my circumstances had suddenly changed. Consequently, Aruna spent the following morning speaking to various colleagues. At the time, she was working as a consultant for the Ontario Ministry of Health. After much negotiating, she arranged for me to be transferred to the geriatric ward of a downtown hospital where a friend of a friend had admitting privileges. The unit itself was the antithesis of the one I was currently on—it was run down and without air-conditioning—but at least it was close to home and my family.

In the meantime, the neurology team had been to see me. They had gathered outside the glass partition that served as the wall between myself and the hallway. I caught snippets of conversation. And telltale phrases leapt out at me: "functional disorder," "conversion reaction," and I even heard "malingering." This last word was most worrisome because it indicated that some of the team proposed that I might be deliberately and consciously contriving my symptoms. From years of experience, I knew that many of them already assumed that I would need to be "taught a lesson."

When they finally entered the room, the lead staff physician didn't even introduce himself and ignored my attempt at extending my hand. (I did my best in such circumstances to preserve my dignity by exhibiting overt goodwill and politeness. It was why I had not complained about my discomfort, weakness, and agitation from my body adjusting to a lack of opiates.) Silent looks passed between them as they watched three young interns undertake a neurological exam of me. One particular test I remember them doing was asking me to raise each leg off the bed while they placed a hand under the opposite leg's heel. I now had some return in my legs, so I could move them, but I couldn't lift them. But I was confused by the hand under my heel—which leg were they examining? I had no idea, but I didn't dare ask. When Aruna visited me later, I asked her about it. She looked a little grim and told me that it was a way of determining whether the weakness and/or paralysis in a leg was organic or functional.[1] Before explaining further, she tested me herself—and then told me, "Well, I read that as organic!"

Regardless, we both grasped that the refusal to treat my pain, the indifference to my opiate withdrawal, the casual response to my call bell, as well as intimations by staff that my symptoms were not real, did not bode well. This hospitalization was not going to be different from most of my previous ones. As such, Aruna sought out the chief resident and told him that she had found a bed in Toronto. The following day I was loaded back into an ambulance for the long drive around Lake Ontario.

To this day, I do not know the real story behind my American hospitalization. Initially, and while in the community hospital in Ithaca, all had gone reasonably well—except for not being able to access the most optimal treatment. But as the weeks wore on, a sense of unease seeped into my care, and it was unclear whether this was due to economic pressures from my health insurance plan or whether the uncertainty about the origin of my paralysis began to disquiet the medical staff. (Interestingly, while I

---

1. The test they used is called "Hoover's sign": if the patient makes involuntary counterpressure with the heel of the one leg while trying to raise the other leg, the leg is likely organically paralyzed.

was in Ithaca, the neurologist there ordered blood tests that were sent to a specialized myasthenia gravis research lab in California, and even though my immune system was being suppressed, I tested positive for one of the "MG antibodies.")

Back in Toronto, I lingered in the dilapidated geriatric wing, awaiting transfer to a rehabilitation unit or hospital—plasmapheresis was out of the question. I very much wanted to go back to the spinal cord/neurological rehab hospital that I had been in a few years earlier. Dr. M., my old physiatrist, was willing to take me, however the rest of her medical team was not prepared to be responsible for someone on myasthenia medications who was not being followed by a neurologist. In the end, after a month or so, I was transferred to a chronic care hospital that was in almost as poor repair as the unit I was leaving.

I stayed six months in this hospital. Again, despite a patient population that was either bedridden or wheelchair bound, none of the bathrooms were accessible. Patients were expected to use bed pans, diapers, or commodes. The lobby, hallways, lounges, and rooms smelled perennially of urine and feces. Because of understaffing of nurses and aides, showers and baths were rationed to once every two weeks—although I managed to negotiate a weekly shower, with a second one to be given by my family (that is, Aruna). Of the two available physiotherapists, one steadfastly refused to treat me because my paresis was "psychological." And, despite my length of stay, I *never* saw my attending physician!

Despite the poor facilities, I worked arduously at improving my strength. My sister-in-law brought me small hand weights to have near my bedside. I used them in the middle of the night when no one could catch me. And very slowly, both time and effort yielded more movement and capacity.

But my family was near disintegration. Our son, Justin, temporarily moved in with his father. I called friends and applied to overnight camps so that our daughter, Alisha, might be distracted and have a carefree summer "away." Aruna's consulting business suffered, and our income dropped precipitously as she spent time with me rather than working. She also had spent every other spare moment looking for a house that either was, or could be made, wheelchair accessible, so that even if I wasn't walking, I could come home. Moreover, as long as I was using a power chair, she could not even take me out in a car. It was only in late summer that I grew strong enough to transfer to and sit in my manual chair.

By Christmas 2000, having narrowly averted bankruptcy (due to the kindness of family and friends who raised money on my behalf) we had found and bought a new house. And, as we began to renovate it to accommodate my wheelchairs, I started to walk with, and then without, crutches—and I came home.

What was more extraordinary was that early in 2001, as movers heaved boxes into our new house, the telephone rang: a university search committee had just short-listed me for a job. A few weeks later, the dean called me with an offer for a tenure-track position at a university in Calgary, near the Rocky Mountains. And so Aruna and I faced one of the bigger decisions of our lives. I felt almost physically ill with the stress. We had each lived in Toronto for almost twenty years; leaving long-established friends and family seemed ludicrous, especially given my dire and unstable health. But the chance to start anew was also seductive. Moreover, I desperately wanted to join the world of my peers and embark on my career. For years, my illness had held me in abeyance, and I often marveled as I watched others writing books, making films, or jetting off to distant cities to make business deals or enjoy holidays. I *yearned* to be a part of that environment. But severing ourselves from all that we knew and from the vibrancy of a city we had truly come to love, wrenched us. Finally, after visiting Calgary with Aruna and the children, we opted to strike out for the West, even as people counseled us that we would inevitably be back.

17 *Gravy*

It has been seven years since we set out westward across the vast expanse of the continent. And many things have changed, but many things also remain the same.

When we first arrived in Calgary, I quickly found a family doctor. Even as I did so, I followed the advice of the pain specialist who had treated me in Toronto. When he knew I was moving, he told me, "Look, I hope you can get a new start there. You have to be truthful about your medical history. But hopefully, they will want to come to your rescue." He chuckled a little, "They'll figure out that the arrogant docs back east screwed up, and they'll want to make up for the mistakes back here." He paused, "So let 'em make us look bad…and I hope you'll get a hell of a lot better care than you have done here—who knows they may even officially diagnose you!"

My new GP was a young woman who was starting her first practice. At our initial meeting, I outlined my illness and the psychogenic diagnosis that had plagued me for over a dozen years. Even as I fretted internally about whether she would kick me out of her office or whether she would even agree to continue prescribing the three or four myasthenia medications I was taking, she seemed to listen to my story without judgment. Instead, we arranged to meet again so that she could give me a physical exam. It was at this appointment that she admitted her lack of experience with neurological symptoms and referred me to neurologist. A couple of weeks later, I told him the same story, and after examining me, he referred me on to the city's neuromuscular clinic, where I have had the same neurologist follow me ever since. As a result, in all the time that I have lived in Calgary, I have not stayed a single night in a hospital—well, that is not entirely true; I stayed up all night sitting at Aruna's bedside after the birth of our youngest son!

But even though the neuromuscular unit follows me, I still do not have an official diagnosis of myasthenia gravis. We've not bothered to replicate the tests that I've had previously in Toronto and elsewhere. We all know that I do not test positive on the single-fiber EMG—the definitive standard for some neurologists—but, we also know that I do react appropriately to Tensilon and that blood tests reveal that I have MG antibodies circulating in my bloodstream. Moreover, I seem to do very well on the treatment protocol for myasthenics even though I do not formally have the disease.

Fortunately, my neurologist continues to prescribe what works. And, because my health has not been stable and I've experienced profound weakness and pain on a chronic basis, he has added drugs and adjusted dosages in an effort to keep my functioning as close to normal as possible. He seems to understand that I have absolutely no desire to be hospitalized and that I want to minimize my symptoms as much as possible. My primary aim is a good quality of life. He thus follows me closely. And, more often than not, the clinic contacts me with a reminder that I am due for my four-month follow-up.

As an occupational therapist and a senior-level health administrator, Aruna is convinced that the fact that I am now a professor gives me more credibility than when I was a very ill graduate student. I suspect that she may be right. Now, instead of having to wait until my breathing stops and I am in extremity, I can simply pick up the phone and be seen by a physician (usually within hours) when I feel unwell or that my strength is faltering. This has meant we have averted the types of crises that would have previously landed me in the ICU and in acute care and then in chronic or rehabilitative care for weeks or months on end.

But, despite this higher standard of care, on a day-to-day basis I still tire very easily. My eyelids droop and my swallowing is permanently compromised. I can't raise my left arm fully and my torso muscles are chronically weak. My joints ache and swell. Typically, one or two symptoms niggle at me at any given time. For example, for the last two months my lower facial muscles have been a little lax. At the beginning of the summer, my mandible hung awkwardly, and I had trouble eating and speaking. My face looked a little expressionless. In fact, my jaw subluxated slightly so that it clicked as I bit down. I tried to spend more time lying down, which sometimes helped and sometimes didn't. More recently, the strength in these muscles seems to be returning—my jaw doesn't feel quite so loose and uncoordinated. The clicking occurs less often. Earlier in the year, my left knee began to catch painfully at different moments—usually as I was transferring weight off the leg. Again, the muscles surrounding the knee and hip were looser than normal. It meant that I was brought up short several times a day as the limb nearly gave out and I had to suppress a yelp of pain. And, as I write this, I have two wound dressings on my feet. The steroids I have used for over a decade have made my skin so fragile that the slightest stretch or impact can open up a crease in my skin; these openings then become easily infected.

I always wear wraparound sunglasses. Students and colleagues often tease me for being "übercool." But I wear them with a purpose. They protect my eyes from harsh light *and* they mask my drooping eyelids from others. This past spring, one of my student evaluations chastised me for falling asleep at the front of the class when I was hosting a guest speaker. I've since realized that I must have forgotten to lower my dark glasses when my eyelids started to collapse. I've also been told that my speech becomes less clear the longer that I lecture; I thus ensure that I wear a lapel microphone in even the smallest of seminars.

My office has a chaise longue so that I can lie down when I am working. I even hold informal meetings from my reclined position on my "couch." If I didn't, I simply wouldn't last more than a day or so before my functioning and strength would become severely compromised. At home, my workstation is in the master bedroom. My bedside table supports stacks of books, files, and papers, and my laptop computer is tucked in a neoprene sleeve by the side of the bed. Invariably I fall asleep with an open pen, and every single one of our sheets and duvet covers has splotches of black or blue ink—much to my own consternation. And, I'm grateful that Aruna seldom complains when she has to slip in beside me, gently nudging papers and folders out of her way.

Currently, I take between thirteen and fifteen medications several times per day—I marvel at my body's ability to absorb and tolerate them. Interestingly, my neurologist added two drugs quite recently that have really helped minimize my physical dips: ephedrine and Lupron. The first we added because I've noticed over the years that I do not falter in the midst of an emergency or stress period; it is afterward that my symptoms roar and I become weak. So as long as adrenaline pumps through me, I am fine; it is when it subsides that I suffer. The ephedrine acts as an artificial adrenaline boost. I take it a couple of times a day. Lupron, the second medication, suppresses my menstrual cycle. We noticed that three to five days per month were very bad for me—I was largely bedridden and in agony—and these days coincided with the three to five days just prior to my period. It also occurred to Aruna and me that *every* time I had had a crisis in the past, I inevitably had a very heavy period the day after landing in ICU. With the aid and advice of an endocrinologist, we turned off my hormonal cycle. Consequently, my "down" days are much less frequent. It has made a substantial and marked difference in my life.

Another key factor in my maintaining my relatively good health has been the fact that I qualify for attendant care under the provincial health plan. My attendant helps me every day and ensures that I do not excessively tire out. Exhaustion is a true enemy, and I have to guard against overexerting myself. I become profoundly weak quite quickly if I place too many demands on myself for a prolonged period of time. This extra bit of assistance makes a substantive difference in my being able to function—without it, I would spend many days a month confined to bed, too weak to see, sit up, or swallow properly.

Overall, we experience much less stress as a family and as a couple knowing that I have access to physicians who treat me with respect and who take my symptoms seriously and respond quickly to anything that may arise. On one occasion, I had to be taken to emergency by ambulance because my doctor thought that I was becoming too weak to stay home. In the ER, Aruna and I were a little surprised by the highly attentive nurse who never left my gurney. Later, the nurse told us that the chief resident had ordered that a member of the crash team remain by me until my breathing stabilized. Thanks to an IV bolus of steroids, retitration of some of my other medications, and morphine for pain, I turned a critical corner and was discharged in the early hours of the following morning. On another occasion, when I was quite weak and ill at home, a visiting nurse took some blood for analysis, and I was diagnosed with acute pancreatitis. Again, I was rushed to the hospital, and again, after concentrated effort, my symptoms subsided. Last autumn, I broke two fingers and a vertebra in my back when I fell. My bone density has diminished as a result of my drug regimen. I unwittingly broke a bone in my foot this summer. Finally, because I am on immune suppressants, every few weeks I fight a chest, sinus, or skin infection that requires antibiotics. We also know that I'm at a higher risk for certain cancers and that I may become diabetic or suddenly go into liver or kidney failure.

Last April, my general practitioner shocked me by saying *aloud* what Aruna and I occasionally said in private and what I had thought many times internally: "Look, you're lucky to be here. Every day that you wake up is gravy—it's a bonus."

We had just weathered a several-month scare in which my blood pressure had risen uncontrollably, my heart showed signs of strain, and blood tests revealed that my kidneys and liver were struggling. The cocktail of drugs was damaging my body. During the early winter, my neurologist proposed a plan to hospitalize me and withdraw all my medications while under medical supervision so that as I gradually lost movement, power, and perhaps, breathing capacity, I could be properly cared for. Further, he began to outline a plan that included a reiteration of all the diagnostic tests I'd had years before. I could sense his resolve to properly diagnose me. Even when I assured him that I would prefer to die moving around from a heart attack or stroke rather than to linger, paralytically, unable to breathe, we were not sure that he was entirely persuaded. What he did make clear was that he could not control his peers who would be on rotation in the neurology unit with him—and, inevitably, I would not always be under his care. Aruna and I were horrified by this prospect. We asked whether he would be willing to restart the treatment protocol for myasthenia gravis even if I did not "test up" properly, and he seemed to equivocate—we sensed that he felt troubled by the difficult political and moral position he might find himself in if this transpired. Knowing that this was a very likely possibility, we realized that, despite the enormous difference in the care I'd received as an outpatient in Calgary, the care I might receive as an inpatient could be overly detached and objective in its insistence on remaining true to defined diagnostic models and to evidence-based medicine (EBM).

In insisting on following only evidence-based practices, clinicians are presumed to provide only those treatments that have substantive evidence or data proving their efficacy. Although in theory this is an extremely good idea and tries to ensure that health care is informed and guided by the latest research, in reality, it does not always work well. In sum, EBM means that patients who are statistical outliers, or who do not meet diagnostically normative models, are potentially overlooked and cannot have their needs met because there is no evidence to back up nonstandard therapies. They do not fit in within a statistical or conceptual framework and thus a clinician cannot back up treatment options with proper scientific evidence.

We were thus very worried that I would once again become acutely vulnerable within a hospital environment that would disbelieve my pain and suffering. To add to our worry, we learned that a woman with myasthenia gravis had suffocated to death while in the proposed hospital when she could not call out or physically indicate her need for help. My neurologist from the neuromuscular clinic tried to allay our fears, stressing that he would admit me to a unit with a lower teaching profile so that there would be fewer hands meddling in my care. But our instincts told us to avoid a hospitalization if at all possible—being an inpatient was too threatening and risky. We pressed for other alternatives.

And, once again, my doctors surprised us. One afternoon, they arranged to meet with Aruna and me to discuss less-drastic options. My neurologist, rheumatologist, endocrinologist, family physician, and several therapists all convened in one room! We collaborated and considered different options. Aruna and I were part of the team, in that our views were validated and considered. In the end, we settled on a plan that included lowering the dosages of some of my medications so that the damage to my internal organs was minimized (or stopped). Even though my body weight could be regarded as normal, I was asked to lose as much as twenty pounds in order to reduce the stress on my heart. And, amazingly, by the spring, everything was different. I had managed to lose ten pounds, and, with a new drug on board and a higher dose of an older one, my blood pressure fell to within normal limits. My EKGs were better. Further, my kidneys and liver had also returned to normal functioning. There was now no need to hospitalize me or back off on my treatment.

Of late, we reconfront the problem of my weak respiration. Strong fatigue, headaches, and blood tests reveal that I am chronically under-oxygenated. On physical exam, my neurologist has noticed that my diaphragm is weaker. The remedy is to try an external ventilator at night so that I am inspiring and exhaling more effectively for at least eight hours a day. We are still uncertain whether I qualify for a prescribed unit under the provincial health plan as my illness differs so enormously from patients who are usually prescribed such devices. With regard to getting the appropriate treatment, my GP, my neurologist, Aruna, and I sense that there may well be clinical, administrative, and financial icebergs ahead. Nonetheless, I have to believe (and hope) that we will navigate them successfully.

I am well enough now to wonder what the significance of this extraordinary journey might be to others. This story of imaginary illness and treatment has been a twenty-year saga. Unless I undergo a miraculous recovery or remission, it will not likely end until I die. I sometimes fantasize about having a bone marrow transplant and having my immune system restarted with stem cells. My hope is that this would "reboot" my defective autoimmune system and allow me to function normally without any need for a concoction of my very damaging medications. But I've learned that this procedure is still experimental and that, much as I like the metaphor of rebooting myself, bone marrow transplants remain highly risky. Moreover, one neuromuscular researcher told me that, since I did not have proper treatment for over a decade, the damage to my nervous and muscular systems is likely permanent and wouldn't necessarily be ameliorated by replacing my immunity. This point has been amply demonstrated when I've met other myasthenic patients who have experienced symptoms for as long as I have (i.e., twenty years) but whose conditions were quickly diagnosed and treated—all of these individuals take no more than one to three medications on any given day and have not experienced lengthy hospitalizations. (By comparison, my fifteen drugs and prolonged hospital stays seem remarkable.)

Despite being unable to return to a beatific existence of health, it is nonetheless very clear that treating my symptoms, even without a formal diagnosis, has quite literally saved my life *and* has saved the health-care system thousands, if not hundreds of thousands, of dollars. As such, I question the efficacy of insisting on disease categories, given that human illness does not usually fit neatly into diagnostic categories. I have yet to meet anyone who has had a textbook case of a disease—individual variations seem to always abound. For example, this past month a friend of mine was hospitalized with viral meningitis—yet it took several days to diagnose her because she also had a (still) unidentified infection in her upper chest. Moreover, her blood work now shows an inexplicably quick recovery to the viral infection but a lingering recovery from the bacteriological one. Another colleague has had serious chronic heart problems for several years, even though his cholesterol and blood pressure remain within the normal range. Even Aruna, when she became pregnant with our last two children, experienced anemia whose origin could not be pinpointed—nor could it be resolved. I could go on and on, reciting a litany of examples of atypical presentations of diseases—they are very common.

As I've shown earlier, disease typing is fairly amorphous. Diseases appear with differing frequencies in differing social, physical, and cultural environments. Diagnostic categories also flex and are adapted as research and clinical experience reveal new information and knowledge about various ailments. Moreover, doctors must understand and apply these paradigms in material contexts that are never ideal—a patient may appear to have a straightforward infection while the clinical picture may be complicated by the patient also having type 1 diabetes, an allergy to penicillin, and having returned from a trip to a tropical rainforest the week before. Consequently, a physician must weigh the probabilities of all these factors in arriving at a diagnosis and a treatment plan. Creating a coherent understanding of what disease process may be going on depends on a range of factors including the doctor's previous clinical experience, textual knowledge, relationships with supervisors, relationships with unit nurses and other allied health professionals, intuitive hunches, and ability to establish a rapport with the patient. Medicine is thus both an objective science and an indefinable art.

Overall, when thinking about my own experience and the problem that diagnosis created for my medical care, I believe that psychogenic theories of disease actually contribute to the reified notion that there are certain illnesses that are "real" and others that are not. It further hardens the perceived divide between mind and body because the clinical response to the psychologizing of disease leads clinicians of all types and professions to blame the patient for his or her symptoms and to view the symptoms as purely the purview of psychiatry. Encounters with nurses and doctors and therapists who vilified me because I was viewed as emotionally unstable taught me that they would not look after me even when I was in extreme physical peril. Moreover, despite nurses often believing themselves to be closer to patients and to be better advocates for their care, I did not find that this was necessarily true. I received good care from any clinician who was able and willing to resist stereotypical beliefs about psychological illnesses.

What is perhaps most frustrating is that the diagnostic definitions of psychogenic illness posit that patients *unconsciously* convert psychological conflicts into physical symptoms; as such, health-care professionals should not view functional illnesses as willful or conscious. But while this may be the theoretical paradigm, clinicians behaved as though I wanted to be ill and that I conspired to confuse and frustrate them. I was treated as though I were a criminal or a juvenile delinquent. Instead of my illness being the problem, *I* became the problem.

Ironically, although I was constantly scrutinized for any and all evidence of psychological abnormalities, this same critical eye was never really turned on any of the clinicians themselves. Confronted by a difficult and ambiguous case, most doctors and nurses routinely grasped for certainty rather than attempting to tolerate any ambivalence. It was easier to categorize me as a "head case" than to accept that I was suffering from an atypical and life-threatening illness about which they had very limited understanding and control. Further, senior members of the medical team often ridiculed the handful of residents, nurses, or therapists who believed me. Clinical hierarchies exerted power over my care that brooked little or no opposition to the official line that my illness and suffering were my own creation and responsibility.

Within this context, my medical chart became a misguided narrative that itemized my bad behavior. It became a way for health-care professionals to flag me as a difficult patient and as way to warn their peers that I undeservedly drained precious medical resources. Computers, faxing, and e-mail facilitated the spread of my poor repute—instead of ameliorating my medical care, these technologies actually contributed to the snowballing of disinformation in my file. It is an appalling fulfillment of the truism about information systems: garbage in, garbage out.

As I became weaker, my capacity to protect myself from any potential hostility in the hospital environment grew less certain. Aruna and I quite literally often wondered whether it would be better to allow me to die than to seek medical assistance. Yet there has been a strong move to "humanize" medicine during the past two decades. And, as part of these reforms, most hospitals have adopted ethics guidelines and committees. But, as a political scientist (who now sits on hospital ethics committees), I have serious reservations about bioethics. I never believed that any "patients' bill of rights"—matted, framed, and hung on a hospital wall—actually protected me when I was sick. I understand that as an adult in a liberal democracy, I enjoy normative rights and equality that transfer into the clinical environment; but I also know that when I am lying in a hospital, paralyzed and incapable of speaking or breathing, that these rights remain abstract and that I'm required to *trust* the physicians, nurses, and therapists who care for me. The problem is that I know that I can't necessarily trust them to look after me! I am haunted by this prospect—that regardless of my legal and ethical status, when I am in a crisis, totally vulnerable and ill, *trust* is my only option. And I can never be sure whether it will be well placed: whether the health professional I encounter will work to ease my psychological and physical suffering and save my life or whether he or she will pay more attention to tests and codified diagnoses. And, even if a clinician does *see* and *believe* me, I don't know whether he or she will be thwarted in his or her efforts on my behalf by others who *distrust* me. So, although one of the motivations behind the adoption of biomedical ethics has been to mitigate the gross power difference between doctors and patients, it seems to me that it has failed to do so, especially in situations of uncertainty and extreme patient debility and vulnerability. I believe that bioethical models have resulted in a template of egalitarian values being superficially slapped over a clinical environment that is both a natural and constructed hierarchy. Sick people are inevitably weaker than those who care for them. And, at the same time, health disciplines remain highly stratified within themselves and in relation to other clinical professions. Biomedical ethics masks these hierarchies from proper scrutiny, evaluation, and critique. And so the hospital will perennially remain a realm of uncertainty and apprehension for me.

However, there is not a day that passes in which I do not feel grateful for the life that I now have. I quite literally have had a second chance at life. Nevertheless, this appreciation is tinged with sadness—sadness that I unnecessarily lost over a decade of my young adulthood to an ailment that could have been properly controlled. This illness has ravaged me physically, psychologically, socially, and economically. The physical costs are obvious, but it was also very difficult to maintain my dignity when so many believed me to be psychologically defective. And my ongoing debility and despair tested my friendships—I lost many of them along the way. Financially, I couldn't work in any real manner until I was thirty-five years old. If I had earned an average salary of $50,000 a year after graduating from college at twenty, it means that I missed out on (at least) $750,000 of income until I became an assistant professor. Moreover, we've paid out very large sums of money for wheelchairs, medical equipment, and accessibility modifications over the two decades. Despite being covered by a universal health-care system and having access to private insurance, many of these expenditures were not covered by health insurance plans because they are seen to be "disability" rather than health-related expenses or else the plans had very low spending caps. Moreover, we know we will likely have more of the same type of expenditures in the future. Thus, even as I enjoy each day that I now live, any contemplation of the past or the future renders unpleasant facts and possibilities that can haunt us, if we let them. There have been losses, and there are likely to be more. On an everyday basis, it's best not to think about them.

Overall, I am incredibly happy. It is amazing what surviving a crucible of experience can yield in terms of emotional health. It has taken a long time for me to realize that, in spite of worries and bumps along the way, I absolutely and totally love life. I feel blissful on most days. I have two grown children who are good, decent, lovely people of whom I am proud and with whom I enjoy spending time. And we also have two more children—two sons, age four and six. And, just as watching Justin and Alisha grow helped sustain me when I was so ill years ago, watching our two young boys now makes me smile several times a day. It also makes me determined that whatever may hit me next (another myasthenic crisis, cancer, heart problems, more broken bones, or the like), I will face them down because I want to raise my youngsters until they are young men. I want and hope to see my children as parents and meet all of my grandchildren one day.

As Canadians, Aruna and I were finally able to marry, eleven years after we met. We are an unorthodox yet typical family of six. But even as I say this, I am very aware that we are a distinct product of our time and place. Medically, if I had been born in an undeveloped area of the world, I would not have had access to the medical knowledge and expertise I required and

I would have long ago been dead. Likewise, if I had been born ten or twenty years earlier, the technological treatments and the pharmaceutical innovations that have both saved and sustained me would not yet have been invented or used. Furthermore, my youngest children wouldn't have been born. And from a sociolegal perspective, if I lived in anything other than a contemporary liberal democracy, I would also not be able to have the family I have now. Less than a hundred years ago, women were not even "persons before the law" in Canada. They could not vote, they could not hold property, and when they worked, their wages were significantly lower than those of their male contemporaries. Here, in Canada, Aruna and I are legally married, and our children are legally both of ours. Moreover, we both hold jobs that we love and that can support our family.

In sum, no matter what the pressures (financial, familial, professional, social, emotional, even medical), my life is *great* as far as I'm concerned. And I'm greedy. I'll take more of it, please—lots more!

Clinical Commentary

BRIAN DAVID HODGES, MD

For any doctor or nurse—anyone whose work is caring for the sick—reading the story of Chloë Atkins's decades' long encounter with the medical system will be as familiar as it is distressing. It certainly was for me. Nonetheless, it has profound resonance with the experiences I have had over the past twenty-five years as a medical student, generalist intern, psychiatry resident, and finally as a professor of psychiatry and medical education. As Atkins's narrative unfolds we meet a cast of characters: some effective, some not; some who convey a sense of warmth and trust, some who are repellant and offensive. As a teacher of many different kinds of health professionals, my thoughts immediately turned to the causes of these variations in professional behaviors. How to explain the stark differences between the doctor who was an "incredibly warm-hearted man, who...tried to treat every patient in the manner he would want his grandmother, mother, or daughter treated" and the one who ordered inappropriate, painful tests to "punish" Atkins? The characters who come off well are few and far between. I am certain that readers who are health professionals will be tempted to dismiss the story, reassuring themselves that it was written by a very unusual patient who has a strange and undiagnosable illness and a life that is complicated by family problems. There will be a temptation for readers, I suspect, to be as dismissive of this narrative as were the clinicians who cared for Atkins. Yet, I hope it is possible to hold on to this discomfort and, rather than turning away, look hard at what Atkins is saying.

In the course of a busy day a doctor, nurse, physiotherapist, or other health professional will see between eight and thirty or more patients in a hospital, community office, or clinic. Some of these people will be charming, clearly presenting their easy-to-fix problems and concluding the interaction with gratitude and certain compliance with the doctor's "orders." Many of these patients will be able to give a complete history, using concise language and accurate descriptions based on their astute observations, complemented by specific details of the effects and side effects of various treatments and medications. Some will have picture-perfect, caring, and supportive families, who attend the appointment, sitting attentively at the patient's side. They will listen carefully to the health-care professional's analysis and dutifully memorize or write down the instructions given, which, on returning home they will conscientiously carry out, perhaps even documenting the effectiveness for the next visit.

Yes, such patients do exist.

However, patients with ill-defined symptoms, difficult-to-diagnose problems, troubled family situations, an inability to give a clear history or to understand information provided to them, and difficulty complying with treatment are, in reality, the norm, not the exception. Illness, disease, and suffering are messy, intense, and profound aspects of human existence that bring forth a full range of emotional complexity and turmoil. They do not always bring out the best in patients. Health professionals, we assume, have the skill to make sense of confusion, shed light where there is darkness, and give hope when there is despair. Atkins's book, then, is about how health professionals work with patients whom they cannot instantly, or perhaps ever, "fix"—those whose presentations are complicated and with whom interaction becomes challenging.

As I sat down to read this chronicle, my first inclination was to sift through the story to try to find Atkins's "real" diagnosis. Does she really have myasthenia gravis? Could it be something else? But, of course, this is the error made by almost everyone whom she encountered. Like all health professionals, I am trained to chase after an explanation, to look for a needle in every haystack, to try to find the one conclusion that will make all of the pieces fall into place. But at some point, we have to step back from the drive to classify and look at the bigger picture. The story Atkins tells is not simply about diagnoses, except perhaps that we should try to turn the lens around and diagnose ourselves and our systems of care.

As I feel when examining a gaping wound, there were times when I wanted to turn away from yet another description of the thoughtless or traumatic care Atkins received. At those moments, it was helpful to remind myself that she, as an author, had the skill to create in me—and in you, the reader—a process akin to what she has experienced her whole life as a patient. Consider how difficult it was for her to delve into the literature on psychosomatic illness—to crack open books and articles filled with the word "psychosomatic," a word that health professionals used again and again to explain away her suffering and sometimes to blame her for it. Yet her confrontation and later mastery of the literature on psychosomatic illness was key to helping her come to terms with her experiences. Through this process she faced some of the demons that stalked her journey through the health-care system and was able to reconcile at a theoretical level some of the ways of thinking that animated the attitudes and approaches of the health professionals she encountered.

Similarly, in reading this narrative, health professionals—indeed anyone with an interest in health care—will inevitably have a similar experience: confrontation with a painful reality that is difficult to ignore. No health professional today with the slightest reflectiveness could fail to notice that patients with highly complex conditions, like those experienced by Atkins, often receive poor care. No one could claim that the management of symptoms in the physical and psychological domains are well integrated. And most health professionals, I hope, have a lingering sense of discomfort when they hear others or themselves speak about individuals as "dumps," "bed-blockers," "nightmare patients," or "frequent-fliers." Fundamentally at odds with an ethos of caring and compassion, this cavalier approach, though sometimes explained away as the pressure valve of "gallows humor," is nevertheless a symptom of a problem of compassion. Atkins's experiences are a call to arms for health-professional educators, and an invaluable text for the study of the relationships between health professionals and patients.

The moving and troubling story that Atkins tells in exquisite detail represents both the justification for and the acute challenge of broadening the frame of competence for health professionals. Time after time, Atkins encountered health professionals who were not skilled at handling interactions with her. Was this a result of training? Of personality? Of the environment in which these individuals studied or worked? Or is there a fundamental problem with the whole enterprise of health professionals and their education? Atkins, while alluding to all of these factors—personality, training, and environment—nevertheless emphasizes the latter: that the diagnostic system of medicine itself is problematic. She decries the Cartesian split of mind and body that erects a wall between physical and psychological explanations and treatments of illness. She also takes aim at the military-like hierarchy that puts the lie to the rhetoric of interprofessional collaboration. Moreover, she thoughtfully shows how the apparently empowering discourse of "patient-centeredness" may actually disguise a darker tendency to shift control and blame onto the individuals who are then "responsible" for the symptoms of their illness.

One of the most astute observations that Atkins makes is that there is a danger when health-care professionals overemphasize the role the individual patient has in taking responsibility for his or her own care. I think there may be a parallel caution needed. We should not overemphasize the role of an individual health professional's responsibility for all the ills of the system. This is particularly true in relationship to the construction of diagnostic categorization itself. Just as the patient is held in objectification by the "medical gaze" so too the student and later the practitioner is shaped, conditioned, and socialized to think and behave within a constrained framework of knowledge and power. As Michel Foucault argued, the use of certain discourses about illness (for example, the idea that there are psychosomatic illnesses) makes it possible to think and say certain things but not others, for health professionals to play certain roles and not others, and for power to accumulate and flow through certain institutions rather than others.

In Atkins's narrative, we see that some of her negative experiences were a product of political, economic, and other factors as much as they were the result of any individual's actions. There is no question that today's health-care environment in Canada, the United States, and in many countries lacks beds, has a shortage of personnel, and struggles with significant financial constraints. While a more political, economic, and sociological view should in no way relieve professionals from the duty to exhibit compassionate and competent behavior, it does draw our attention to the way the context in which health professionals, patients, and their families interact contributes to problems. As the University of Toronto, Department of Pediatrics professor Tina Martimianakis has written, "a focus on individual characteristics and behaviours alone is insufficient as a basis on which to build further understanding of professionalism and represents a shaky foundation for the development of [health professional] educational programmes and tools."[1] For these reasons I have focused on Atkins's narrative at two different levels: that of the individual health professional, and that of the health-care education system.

There are many lessons to be learned from this story. I will address four:

1. Diagnosis and classification—the changing constructions of illness
2. The mind-body conundrum
3. Empathy and dignity—the objectification of diseases rather than patients
4. Lessons for health-professional education

Diagnosis and Classification—the Changing Constructions of Illness

What Is Diagnosis?

Whether we trace the origin of medicine to Hippocrates' lectures about bodily humors given under a plane tree in ancient Greece, to Chinese

---

1. Martimianakis, M. A., Maniate, J., Hodges, B. D. (2009). "Sociological Interpretations of Professionalism." *Medical Education* 43, no. 9 (Sept.): 829–37.

physicians who, thousands of years ago, described a system of meridians and energy flow, or to Arabic physicians who developed many of the first effective treatments, we can see that diagnosis has been an overarching concern in the field that we group together in the flexible category called "medicine." Diagnosis is, as Atkins writes in this book, "an attempt to impose order and coherency on apparently random physiological events." Indeed, it has been said that in the face of uncertainty, humankind's first response is categorization. However, as soon as we categorize, we lump together things that are similar but not the same. In doing so, we lose some of the richness of the original conditions. It is sometimes assumed that a diagnostic label implies a known and unified conceptual mechanism that explains all similar "cases" and that medical diagnoses are inherent and stable categories of human illness. However, a review of medical history and sociology makes it evident that quite the opposite is true; disease categories are highly unstable and reflect the dominant and changing theories and discourse of the time. As Atkins observes, "through the centuries, medicine has employed a variety of frameworks with which to understand the human body and its illnesses (humoral, germ theory, etc). Society, culture, and technology influence the construction and reconstruction of disease in both time and place." Let us consider a contemporary example. When I was in medical school in the late 1980s, we spent a whole week studying the factors that were believed to cause gastric ulcer. The gastroenterologists gave us detailed explanations of how life stressors and personality factors led to the red, eroded, and angry pathological stomach tissue that we could view in the laboratory. This was my understanding of gastric ulcer until 2005 when the Nobel Prize for medicine was awarded to the Australian professors Barry J. Marshall and J. Robin Warren, whose twenty-five-year-old discovery that a major cause of gastric ulcer was a bacteria and that treatment with an antibiotic was most effective finally came to be accepted.[2] This 180-degree turn echoed, almost one hundred years later, a lesson from the work of

2. Marshall, B. J., Warren, J. R. (1984). "Unidentified Curved Bacilli in the Stomach Patients with Gastritis and Peptic Ulceration." *Lancet* 1, no. 8390: 1311–15.

Dr. Paul Ehrlich, the 1908 Nobel Prize winner who discovered that *tabes dorsalis,* a paralytic and dementing condition that confined crippled and intellectually diminished victims to asylums in the nineteenth century, was in fact caused by the syphilis spirochete.

This is not to suggest that all diseases will eventually be found to have an infectious cause, or even that we can hope to find the "real" cause of all symptom clusters, illnesses, and diseases. It is to argue, however, that those who wield the power of diagnosis must do so with humility. Moliere's classic comedy *Le malade imaginaire* (*The Imaginary Invalid*) is a scathing critique of the overconfidence of seventeenth-century physicians who treated patients with emetics and bloodletting based on the ancient Greek theory of humors and ignoring evidence that blood circulated in the veins, something proven decades earlier by William Harvey.[3] In fact, when the cause of an illness is vague or speculative, popular discourses (ways of thinking and speaking) of the time and place become associated in an explanatory way with symptoms.[4] For example, in nineteenth-century England and America, when the nervous system was being discovered, patients and their doctors tended to attribute symptoms of poorly understood conditions to "neurasthenia," a presumed neurological incapacity. Later, in the early twentieth century with the rise of Freudian thought, explanations of the mind and psychosexual conflict made diagnoses such as "hysteria" common. In the late twentieth century, when there was greater interest in the immune system and more attention to the environment, in the face of uncertainty more explanations became linked to immune dysfunctions and environmental causes.

I am quite certain that there are neurological, immunological, psychological, and environmental explanations for many of the signs, symptoms, and behaviors experienced by patients today. However, we must

---

3. Molière (Jean-Baptiste Poquelin). (1997/1673). *Le malade imaginaire.* Paris: Larousse-Bordas.

4. Shorter, E. (1992). *From Paralysis to Fatigue: A History of Psychosomatic Illness in the Modern Era.* New York: Maxwell Macmillan International.

also remain vigilant that we do not put the diagnostic cart too far in front of the evidence horse. Even in domains where medicine presumes to be standing on firm diagnostic ground, caution is required. How many people, physicians included, appreciate that the most common presentation of myocardial infarction (heart attack) in women is *not* chest pain but rather lethargy? Or that when doctors discover abnormal findings on an ECG they are more likely to interpret a cardiac cause in men than in women?[5] Decades of studies conducted almost exclusively on white, middle-aged, Euro-American men means that even our "solid ground" is built on highly selective evidence.[6]

Please Diagnose Me with Something

Given all of the caveats and cautions noted above, one might wonder why a clinician would ever venture to make a diagnosis in the face of ambiguity. And one may also wonder why patients so desperately want to be diagnosed with "something." Indeed, in clinical situations I feel a great reluctance to articulate or write a diagnosis in a chart until I have reached a degree of certainty. Many conditions can never be proven with certainty in life (for example, the neurological findings of Alzheimer's usually cannot be shown until autopsy) if ever (there are no conclusive diagnostic tests for autism or schizophrenia). Yet providing a diagnosis helps to structure the approach of health professionals. Having a diagnosis in mind makes it easier to access specific knowledge about the condition and engage in a treatment plan. It is difficult to describe how uncomfortable we physicians feel when we have no idea what is wrong with a patient.

For patients, too, diagnosis gives meaning and provides order. Which is why Atkins so desperately wanted one—one that was physical, that is. To have a diagnosis is to have a vision of what one is up against, no matter

5. McSweeney, J. C., Cody, M., O'Sullivan, P., Elberson, K., Moser, D. K., Garvin, B. J. (2003). "Women's Early Warning Symptoms of Acute Myocardial Infarction." *Circulation* 108:2619–23.

6. Phillips, S. (1995). "The Social Context of Women's Health: Goals and Objectives for Medical Education." *Can Med Assoc J* 152, no. 4: 507–11.

how terrible the possible future: "Better the devil you know then a devil you don't know." Enduring a long period when one's diagnosis is uncertain can be a painful and frustrating experience. Even when a doctor only "suspects" something, patients and families want to know what it is. As Atkins writes, "the stability of disease typing provides tremendous benefit to both the ill individual and the physician.... Hopes and fears are focused on a tangible entity. Together the lay person and the practitioner attempt to resolve the amorphous void of illness and replace it with the clearer certainty of disease." We see a good example of this shared benefit when, on a visit to Montreal, Atkins and her partner speak of a "suspected" diagnosis of myasthenia gravis, the health professionals confidently undertake a predetermined series of clinical acts.

Interestingly, disclosure of diagnosis is an area of professional practice that has changed substantially over my career. Less than twenty years ago when I was in medical school, we were taught that the treatment team might wish to withhold the diagnosis from a dying patient lest the truth lead him or her to lose hope and die sooner. Today, withholding the truth from patients and families is considered unprofessional behavior and relegated to an outmoded and paternalistic past. In the same vein, a common practice in the midtwentieth century was for a physician to discuss a woman's illness with her husband. Today this would smack of a paternalistic breach of confidentiality. Yet these changes, which have taken place in just a few decades, cannot be explained simply by the advancement of medical science. Rather, professional norms also change as a result of shifting social values. What practices are in play today that will seem archaic a few years hence? I suspect that the influence of migrants from countries where the doctor is expected to conduct interactions with the whole family—never with the individual alone—will further challenge and modify our understanding of what constitutes appropriate "disclosure." For the moment, a thorough and frank discussion of the "differential diagnosis" with the individual patient who is struggling with the illness is the norm. With the exception of a few patients who insist that they "don't want to know," talking about diagnosis and treatment increases understanding, reduces anxiety, and can provide a mechanism by which the doctor and patient affirm a shared commitment to tackle the illness. As Atkins writes, "on the one hand, I wanted to be well regardless of the diagnosis. On the other, I wanted to have a specific disease—an entity that could be identified, named, and treated. If I had no diagnosis, then my symptoms meant nothing."

However, for the doctor and patient (and possibly the family) to have such a discussion, all of the information must be on the table. It is not sufficient for a physician simply to state what the diagnosis is (or might be). When I teach first-year medical students communications skills, one of the first things I tell them is that they must know what the *patient* thinks the explanation for their symptoms might be. As Atkins points out, "practitioners and patients form a symbiotic relationship in which the meaning and significance of a disease can be easily understood and accepted by both parties." Medical students are initially confused and surprised when I tell them that a diagnosis is not a fixed entity—but rather a product of the scientific, social, economic, and cultural milieu in which both the doctor and patient exist: it is a shared creation. I often use cross-cultural examples to illustrate this. To cite only one, if a patient's understanding of their low energy level involves the flow of qi through their meridians and the doctor's understanding is that the symptom results from a lack of neurotransmitters in the brain, it will take a few conversations to see if common ground can be found, or at least to establish that the doctor and patient will work within more than one paradigm. In Atkins's narrative, we see that this common ground was rarely found. Atkins observes that "doctors insisted that I was unconsciously (and some even believed consciously) making myself ill....I became the embodiment of an ancient Greek paradigm of hysteria...for which no organic cause can be found." Clearly, this was not the explanation that she held for her suffering. She observes that "most people would be happy to discover that 'there's nothing wrong with you.'" However, what she was actually being told was *not* that nothing was wrong with her but rather (often indirectly) that there *was* something was wrong with her, but that the something was *a product of her own mind.*

The Mind-Body Conundrum

The Legacy of Decartes

I have worked in the space between physical and psychological medicine for many years, and Atkins has done an excellent job of reviewing the history and literature of the mind-body conundrum. Medicine has struggled with and will continue to struggle with the twists and turns of what we call "psychosomatic medicine." As Atkins points out, the essence of this field is "the extraordinary and incalculable interpenetration of the mind and body." For centuries anyone with an interest in human suffering has been aware that no explanation of human physical disease is complete without including the mind. It is normative in our society to accept, for example, that worry and stress can make a person ill or exacerbate an existing condition. It is widely known that there are connections between anger, blood pressure, and heart disease; between hope and recovery from cancer; between stress and infectious diseases. More formally, science has helped us to understand the "placebo effect," a mechanism whereby the simple belief in the pill one is given can lead to impressive treatment effects, even when the medication is chemically inert. Similarly, physical symptoms such as pain and fatigue can have a profound effect on one's mood, concentration, and ability to think and process information.

Since the early twentieth century, behavioral theories have helped us understand that the body and mind can work together in ways that are not usually evident. Studies of "biofeedback" and of Eastern traditions of yoga and meditation show clearly that one can learn to control basic biological functions such as heart rate, blood pressure, and even pain. In her narrative, Atkins notes this interplay of her mind and body. She writes, "I know that pain thins my concentration and makes me irritable." She also describes the role that depression had in reducing her capacity to endure physical symptoms, that she experienced "intense migraines from the stress of appearing congenial while feeling completely helpless, silenced, terrified, and alone." While there is little doubt about a strong interplay of mind and body, Atkins's experiences illustrate major problems with the way this interplay is enacted in today's health-care system.

First there is the legacy of the seventeenth-century French philosopher René Descartes, who is credited with (and blamed for) describing the mind-body divide that still plagues Western thinking. As Atkins rightly points out, "the Cartesian divide between the mind and the body remains rigidly in place in hospitals," meaning that significant effort is expended to determine if a symptom is a product of the body (called "organic") or the mind (called "functional"). The result of making an either/or determination is that, rather than serving to integrate the two parts into a diagnostic and treatment whole, a sort of diagnostic triage leads a patient either to a physical specialist (neurology, internal medicine, etc.) or a psychological one (psychiatry, psychology, etc.). While there are specialties that attempt to bridge this divide (geriatrics, palliative medicine, pain medicine, and my own specialty of consultation-liaison psychiatry), Atkins is right in observing that the underlying *thinking* sustains the dichotomy. Hospitals increasingly employ the services of consulting psychiatrists and psychologists for patients with psychological symptoms, but other health-care professionals remain quite intolerant of anything for which they cannot find a hard "organic" cause. Conversely, I have been amazed over my years of practice how resistant psychiatric units are to admitting patients with a physical illness, refusing to transfer anyone until they are "medically clear" (a concept that is as unhelpful as it is unrealistic), and the rarity of my colleagues attempting even a perfunctory physical examination.

The result of this persistent mind-body split is the use of a "psychological/functional" category reserved for conditions for which no *other* explanation can be found. This renders psychosomatic illnesses "diagnoses of exclusion"—diagnoses that are left when everything else is eliminated. The binary of organic versus functional illness is further reinforced when a patient arrives in a hospital unit that gives little if any consideration to the other part of the binary. Yet research shows that significant psychological dimensions are present in most, if not all, patient presentations and that many patients with psychological symptoms also have physical diseases. I agree with Atkins when she says that "even though neurologists and psychiatrists both deal with diseases of the mind/brain, the divide between the two fields remains strong" and that "there may be new psychological discourses about illness, but the actual arrangement of specialties means that physicians are really ill-equipped to respond to patients in a truly holistic manner." The result is, as Atkins notes, that people often leave a doctor's office with a diagnosis of stress-related or psychogenic illness but that "these categories do not necessarily help the patient get better."

"Behavior" Is Not a Symptom

A second problem is how professionals approach patients who exhibit complex behaviors associated with an illness. Atkins recognized the role that she could play, albeit with limited effectiveness, in modifying her behavior. She described, for example, her efforts at "coaching myself to draw more [breath] deeply and with greater frequency." However, the many doctors, nurses, and therapists she depended on lacked the skill to recognize and appropriately separate out the contribution and malleability of behavioral dimensions of her illness. While nurses, in particular, and some physicians used the epithet "behavior" to denote something volitional and primarily undesirable, behavior is actually a very complex symptom. Health professionals demonstrate serious confusion about which behaviors are acceptable symptoms of illness (involuntary movements, unusual speech inflections, and vocalizations); which are partially voluntary but warrant attention and therefore are seen as symptoms (suicide attempts, self-harm); and which are simply *bad behavior* (complaining, signing out of hospital against medical advice, noncompliance with treatment).

This issue is thrown into sharp relief, when, relatively early in her experience, Atkins deliberately infected an IV line. I remember my shock when, as an intern, I discovered that a patient who displayed all the signs and symptoms of acute kidney stones was actually pricking his finger and putting blood into his urine bottle. From that day forth, what I needed to do, and what all health professionals need to do, was look beyond the feelings immediately induced by such events and ask probing questions of the patient (and of ourselves) that aim at understanding rather than blame. What does the health professional do when such an event raises strong emotions? If the first reaction is one of fear, dread, anger, or another strong emotion, the best approach is to go for a short walk (see the heading "Everyone's Judgment Is Compromised Sometimes"). As soon as possible, however, it is important to further investigate the situation with the same steady calm and curiosity that one would bring to asking about any other event, be it an accident, a heart attack, or a fainting spell. The situation should be acknowledged directly, but with a tone of curiosity, not of judgment: "I would like to understand what led to the situation in which you felt you needed to put your own blood in your urine [or infect your own IV]." The interrogation needs to be about the patient's behavior certainly, but also about the circumstances. Why would someone do such a thing? The health professional must keep in mind a broad formulation of the behavior: To what is it attributable? Could it be confusion or mental illness? Could it be an intentional manipulation (for insurance reasons for example)? Or perhaps the patient was feeling abandoned and simply trying to get help? The goal is to understand, with the patient's help, what such an act means. Categories such as factitious disorder, conversion disorder, or Munchausen syndrome—disorders in which unusual physical symptoms are assumed to have psychological origins—are often used to dismiss patients from care rather than engaging them in treatment.

Over and over again, as they worked with Atkins, health professionals made a key error. Even if she might have been able to learn behavioral control over some biological functions (for example, the physical control of breathing during intubation is sometimes possible, if difficult) Atkins's health professionals appear not to have known how to help her with this. Why? Because behavioral modification is difficult and takes practice. It is striking that, on the one hand, her therapists acknowledged that to gain function in a limb, Atkins would have to undergo a painstaking, continuous, and repeated regimen of physiotherapy, while, on the other, they assumed that she could gain control over her breathing if they simply yelled at her. Clearly the physicians and other health professionals Atkins encountered believed that she could control some of her behavioral symptoms. However, they never asked, "Do you believe you have any control over your breathing/movement/gait? If so, in what ways and under what circumstances?"

As I described above, biofeedback has taught us that humans can gain control over many bodily functions including respiration, heart rate, and even blood pressure. We all have some control that can be accessed through training. We can learn to control the mind-body link. I spent many years helping patients who experienced panic attacks learn conscious control over bodily functions such as breathing and heart rate. But such treatment does not take place in an afternoon. Rather, this ability to control symptoms and behaviors only begins to occur after the tenth or fifteenth session of coaching, exercises, and learning such things as "box breathing," a technique that prevents hyperventilation. Then the patient can make an initial visit to a train station or a shopping center (or whatever triggers a panic attack for the individual). And that will be a point of further departure, not the end of the journey.

This systematic approach was entirely lacking in the care Atkins received. Her behavioral symptoms induced such antipathy in health professionals that a behavioral approach to complement physical investigations and treatments was never considered. This is unfortunate because behavioral interventions can be undertaken even in the intensive care unit. The appropriate use of such techniques, however, takes as much training and competence as putting in an intravenous line or performing a lumbar puncture. In the absence of specific training, the professionals in the various hospitals and clinics she visited adopted only half of the behavioral paradigm. That is, they accepted that human bodily functions could be voluntarily controlled but ignored that learning to do so is a complex and inevitably incomplete process that requires deliberate practice in the presence of a skilled and competent coach.

All of which leads to questions about the behavior of health professionals. As a doctor, I need to understand that *my* behavior is important. I cannot simply order patients to take their medications or to follow instructions and hope that they will all do so in a timely and effective manner. Human behavior is complex. In learning to be a doctor, I had to learn to understand and use encouragement, to convey hope and to adopt the rallying spirit of a coach. Doctors and nurses also need to learn to wield with ethical thoughtfulness the placebo effect, while ever vigilant for the appearance of its evil twin—"nocebo."[7] The nocebo effect occurs when a negative or harmful outcome occurs merely because it was suggested, even though the treatment was inert. Health professionals frequently induce such negative self-fulfilling prophecies without awareness of the power of their words and attitudes.

If we are to effectively care for the sick, we need to understand that there is a profound, problematic split in the conceptualization of illness and in the organization of health-care delivery that perpetuates a separation of mind and body. However, while the diagnostic classification and organization of health-care institutions and professions is problematic, the attitude and interpersonal skills of individual health professionals are even more germane to the experiences of patients. Atkins writes, "I received good care from any clinician who was able and willing to resist the stereotypical beliefs about psychological illness." While philosophical, sociological, and systems aspects of health care may be a little abstract for students learning to be health professionals, or even for their teachers, the attitudes and skills of communication, collaboration, and advocacy are not.

Empathy and Dignity: The Objectification of Diseases Rather than Patients

Objectifying the Patient

Medical educators in North America, in particular, since the 1980s, have greatly increased the curricular time devoted to teaching communication and interpersonal skills. Indeed, research has shown that good communication skills are linked strongly to improved treatment outcomes,[8] increased compliance with medical recommendations,[9]

7. Barsky, A. J., Saintfort, R., Rogers, M. P., Borus, J. F. (2002). "Nonspecific Medication Side Effects and the Nocebo Phenomenon." *JAMA* 287, no. 5 (Feb. 6): 622–27.

8. Di Blasi, Z., Harkness, E., Ernst, E., Georgiou, A., Kleijnen, J. (2001). "Influence of Context Effects on Health Outcomes: A Systematic Review." *Lancet* 357:757–62.

9. Vermeire, E., Hearnshaw, H., Van Royen, P., Denekens, J. (2001). "Patient Adherence to Treatment: Three Decades of Research—A Comprehensive Review." *J Clin Pharm Ther*

decreased pain,[10] reduced recovery time,[11] increased patient satisfaction,[12] and decreased medical litigation.[13] Today, when we teach communication skills in medical school we often start by talking about problems with the way physicians were trained in the late nineteenth to mid-twentieth century. In those days large teams of white-coated physicians (mostly men until the late twentieth century) conducted "rounds" by moving herdlike from bed to bed, discussing signs, symptoms, and diagnoses with one another but without ever involving the patient. In my training I remember senior physicians who asked me to demonstrate physical examination techniques or interesting pathological findings on patients without even saying hello to the patient or introducing the members of the team. This rendered the patient a silent object that the team scrutinized and examined. I use the past tense in my description because this mode of teaching is supposed to have fallen out of favor. Ideally, what some call "patient-centered care" has replaced objectification with interactions that *involve* the patient.

However, rendering patients as "objects" for examination through what Foucault called "the medical gaze" remains a powerful dynamic in medicine and a common occurrence in medical education. Despite efforts to humanize teaching rounds, the health-care environment remains replete with objectification. This is why Atkins often felt that "people rushed by

26:331–42. Kim, S. S., Kaplowitz, S., Johnston, M. V. (2004). "The Effects of Physician Empathy on Patient Satisfaction and Compliance." *Eval Health Prof* 27:237–51.

10. Berk, S. N., Moore, M. E., Resnick, J. H. (1977). "Psychosocial Factors as Mediators of Acupuncture Therapy." *J Consult Clin Psychol* 45:612–19.

11. Thomas, M. R., Dyrbye, L. N., Huntington, J. L., Lawson, K. L., Novotny, P. J., Sloan, J. A., Shanafelt, T. D. (2007). "How Do Distress and Well-Being Relate to Medical Student Empathy? A Multicenter Study." *J Gen Intern Med* 22:177–83.

12. Bertakis, K. D., Roter, D., Putnam, S. M. (1991). "The Relationship of Physician Medical Interview Style to Patient Satisfaction." *J Fam Pract* 32:175–81. Donovan, J. L. (1995). "Patient Decision-Making: The Missing Ingredient in Compliance Research." *Int J Technol Assess Health Care* 11:443–55.

13. Levinson, W. (1994). "Physician-Patient Communication: A Key to Malpractice Prevention." *JAMA* 272:1619–20. Beckman, H. B., Markakis, K. M., Suchman, A. L., Frankel, R. M. (1994). "The Doctor-Patient Relationship and Malpractice: Lessons from Plaintiff Depositions." *Arch Intern Med* 154:1365–70.

us as though we were furniture." In a busy ward or clinic, health professionals are often so focused on the tasks at hand that they forget to interact with patients and families. Not long ago, as I was making my way back to my hospital office from the coffee shop, I passed by the radiology department. Clutching my coffee, I passed the rows of seats filled with patients waiting in the busy hallway for an X-ray. Just as I turned the corner to leave the department, a technician called out, "Is the two o'clock pelvis here yet?"

Talking about patients as body parts (e.g., "the liver in 212," "the double lung admitted yesterday"), as diseases ("the schizophrenic," "the epileptic") or as cases ("the fracture in 309") is part of the objectification process. The "chart" further reinforces the objectification of patients because this historical document often stands in for, or even supplants, what a patient has to say. Of course, having access to a patient's chart is invaluable for health professionals because it documents past treatments and responses, allergies and medications—details that are often vague or unremembered by patients and families. But as we see repeatedly in Atkins's narrative, the arrival of the chart with its labels, analyses, and opinions given by others in the past can change completely the attitudes of a team of health professionals. I recall many times trying to find a bed for a patient I had seen in my emergency department, knowing that my description to colleagues over the phone would have to be very convincing to counter words like "borderline personality disorder," "chronically suicidal," or "acts out" that could be found in the chart. I know that as soon as my colleagues read words such as "difficult patient" or "noncompliant" their attitude will change, and the likelihood that they will take an empathic stance will diminish.

Of course, sometimes knowing that patients have had difficulties in the past can be helpful. Some conditions and behaviors do actually get worse in hospital settings. For example, a patient who has tried to cut himself or herself repeatedly but who is not harboring suicidal thoughts may gain more from supportive outpatient care than from admission to a highly charged inpatient psychiatric unit where interaction with other distressed patients can aggravate the problem. Similarly, it is helpful to know that a patient has a history of being violent, of leaving unannounced, or becoming threatening so that proactive steps can be taken to anticipate and minimize these events. However, such written (and frequently indirect or "coded") communications strongly shape the way health professionals listen to and interpret patients' situations and symptoms and are helpful to the patient only if clinicians are prepared to adapt their approach to help the "difficult" or "noncompliant" patient.

In his book *How Doctors Think* Jerome Groopman touched on these issues, though he avoided an in-depth discussion of specifically psychological aspects of the doctor-patient relationship. He noted that he does not write about psychiatry because it is a different context and its practitioners have a unique way of thinking. It seems to me that this may be a symptom of the separation of "mind" and "body" medicine that I described above. However, the book does provide useful tips to help patients focus their stories and ask pointed questions, and to consider second and third opinions. Nevertheless, patients who have read the book tell me that beyond organizational and linguistic strategies, it is difficult for them to adapt to situations in which the problem is a fundamental lack of empathy on the part of health-care professionals. It might be said that *How Doctors Think* subtly conveys the message that the way doctors think is not likely to change and that patients would be wise to learn to adapt to it. I would argue the converse: that the way doctors think should, in some cases, change.

Atkins's narrative illustrates why the ability to convey empathy and attend to patient dignity remains an underemphasized competence for today's health professionals. As a physician, I have a responsibility to understand, not just a patient's anatomy and physiology, but also how she or he thinks and feels. This is just as true for nurses, physical therapists, and occupational therapists, nutritionists, pharmacists, and all in the health professions. Certainly, as Groopman and others have written, it is helpful for patients to learn strategies to adapt to the thoughts, behaviors, and practices of health professionals. And there is no question that it can be helpful for patients and families to read about their problems on the Internet. But, surely, doctors and other health professionals need to also understand and adapt to *how patients think.*

How do patients think? What do patients want? I suspect that many health professionals have never asked. Here Atkins gives us a glimpse of some things that many patients want. Patients don't want to feel judged. They want someone who listens to them. They appreciate it when, even if nothing else can be done, someone says, "I am sorry this is happening to you. I don't know what it is, but I am going to try to help you figure it out."

Empathy

The idea that health professionals engage with patients through understanding their worldviews, values, and interests is known as empathy.[14] Indeed, Atkins greatly valued the clinicians who tried to see things from her perspective, those who "always treated me with respect and continued to ponder the possibility that my illness was, indeed, 'real.'" It is hard work to be empathic. I find it difficult when I am tired, frustrated by a situation, or anxious about a diagnosis or treatment situation. Indeed, there is a robust literature that shows that empathy declines in medical students as their training advances, as they develop something called "detached concern."[15] However, I try to remember, and to remind my students, that we health professionals can become far too detached and that in the most difficult situations a few well-chosen words can change the nature of the therapeutic relationship. I have taught communication skills to medical and other health-professions students for many years and find that the concept of "empathy" is rather nebulous for students. Thus it may be more useful to examine closely some of the characters in Atkins's narrative and pick apart the specific approaches and behaviors that made some of them more effective than others. These elements include engaging the patient and attending to emotional reactions; being curious and thinking broadly; and preserving dignity and establishing trust.

14. Yarascavitch, C., Regehr, G., Hodges, B. D., Haas, D. A. (2009). "Changes in Dental Student Empathy during Training." *J Dent Educ* 73, no. 4 (April): 509–17.

15. Spencer, J. (2004). "Decline in Empathy in Medical Education: How Can We Stop the Rot?" *Med Educ* 38: 916–18.

Engaging the Patient and Attending to Emotional Reactions

I suspect that if we could interview the health-care professionals who encountered Atkins, some might tell us that they did not "like" her. Atkins herself notes that the weight of her illness, the seesawing distress of an undiagnosed condition, and a heavy overlay of psychological stress "burned people out." In her words, "I appeared narcissistic and self-preoccupied—which I was." But is likeability a precondition for caring? To use a little medical jargon, many patients "regress" to a "sick role" when they are overtaken by illness. We all experience this sick role when we have a flu or fever and retreat passively to bed and are appreciative when a friend or family member nurtures us back to health. If we are sicker than that, we become anxious, frightened, irritable, even angry. This sick role is well tolerated by others with certain restrictions: that the illness has a clear cause, that it is of short duration, and that the patient bounces back to good health. If these criteria are not met, as in the case of chronic health problems, friends and family may disengage or even become hostile. While health professionals can become affected by the same reactions, it is much less appropriate in the professional sphere, where the goal should be to engage with all patients, no matter how complex or difficult their presenting problems are.

Lest the reader conclude, as do some students in the health professions, that all of this talk of empathy is simply about "being nice," I should like to provide an important nuance. While being respectful and preserving patient dignity is essential to all patient encounters, there are times when empathy can be shown in ways that might not be construed as "nice." In fact, an overly passive health professional may not foster the sense of confidence needed for a patient to overcome obstacles, such as a difficult rehabilitation. I have seen many patients who are struggling to breathe on their own so that staff can remove their ventilator, a terrifying event that Atkins portrays skillfully in her narrative. Simply being nice to someone undergoing this struggle is not, however, particularly helpful. While one must be supportive, understanding, and prepared to tolerate failures and setbacks, it is most useful to help patients set goals and strongly encourage them to reach them—much like a coach with an athlete.

An engaged approach is nicely illustrated early in Atkins's narrative when she describes an occupational therapist who, though we would probably not call her "nice," nevertheless employed firmness combined with patience that allowed Atkins to find her limits and challenge them, while continuously encouraging progress. Her surprisingly blunt style ("Stop being embarrassed!") was nevertheless effective because she simultaneously "gave hope" and acknowledged "potential disappointment." And of, course, there will be times when health professionals do not agree with patients or families, when they have different understandings or values that cannot be reconciled or when there are insurmountable systems issues (availability of resources, treatments, etc.). In my experience, these can nevertheless be dealt with when there is an underlying sense of engagement between the patient and the health-care team.

Certainly, it is easier to engage with people whom we like. However, being a professional—as opposed to family member or friend—means taking care of people you don't know. The hallmark of professional competence is to be able to care for people who are difficult, who are unlikable, who cannot be easily engaged. In several instances that Atkins recounts, lack of skill in helpful engagement led to hostility and anger that were unhelpful to the patient and her health professionals. In fact, rather than there being helpful engagement, both patient and professionals disengaged completely. The potential for such disengagement is so strong that we must learn strategies to deal with it. I suggest to students that when they feel hostility or anger toward a patient they should reflect on the causes. Blaming a patient for his or her own illness is a clue that the health professional is feeling helpless or frustrated. If he or she becomes angry an important diagnostic and therapeutic opportunity may be missed. The skilled health professional asks himself or herself *why* they are becoming angry or dismissive. A phenomenon at the base of this is often "projective identification"—a mechanism whereby a doctor or nurse absorbs and experiences similar feelings to that which a patient is experiencing. We all recognize that emotions are infectious, and that when we are at the bedside with someone sad, we may feel a bit sad after we leave. What is less well understood is that we have the same capacity to "absorb" other emotions—frustration, helplessness, even anger, and reflect them back to the patient.

A wonderful illustration of the importance of attending to such emotions comes from the research of Dr. Roger Kneebone at Imperial College in London.[16] Dr. Kneebone trains medical students to perform routine procedures such as giving injections and starting an IV on plastic models, as is common in medical schools around the world. However Dr. Kneebone's clever innovation is to mount the plastic model on a real person: an actor, who plays the part of a patient. Dr. Kneebone and his team train these "simulated patients" to have additional problems such as anger or confusion. The research results are dramatic. Medical students who regularly ask calm and compliant patients about a penicillin allergy before giving an injection often "forget" to ask when the patient is angry, forging ahead with the dangerous injection. For others, facing a hostile or confused patient results in a dramatic reduction of their ability to take a history. The research shows clearly that when an emotional aspect is added to doctor-patient encounters of various kinds it alters everything from doctors' thinking to their ability to carry out technical skills. Thus, awareness and mastery of one's emotions are criteria for competence in health professionals and key requirements for engagement with patients. Competent health professionals attend to their own feelings and try to understand what they mean, while incompetent health professionals dismiss their own emotions and in the process disengage from their patients.

Being Curious and Thinking Broadly

Curiosity is another attribute that separates professionals who engage with patients in helpful and therapeutic ways from those who becomes angry or dismissive. In Atkins's narrative we see signs that some health professionals became curious rather than angry. For example, she

16. Kneebone, R., Bello, F., Nestel, D., Yadollahi, F., Darzi, A. (2007). "Training and Assessment of Procedural Skills in Context Using an Integrated Procedural Performance Instrument (IPPI)". *Stud Health Technol Inform* 125:229–31.

describes a nurse who approached her "with a mixture of regret and concern.... I could see that my situation puzzled her"; there was a doctor who "seemed to intuit my concerns"; there was a family doctor in Calgary who could "listen to my story without judgment." Once the health professional is curious about a patient's problems, it is easier to focus on the question, how can I be helpful to this person?

How do. we foster curiosity in health-care settings when it is absent? For students, learning to create a "bio-psycho-social" formulation is a core competence that helps to see patients' presenting problems from different angles. In such a formulation, the biological, psychological, and social predisposing, precipitating, and perpetuating factors are all identified, and the interplay between different domains is considered. For example, imagine a middle-aged woman who presents with a heart attack. The predisposing factors may be biological (hypertension), behavioral (smoking), psychological (depression leading to inactivity), and social (poverty leading to poor diet, inability to afford treatment, exposure to poor environment, social isolation) all at once. No single factor can, or should, be given too much or too little consideration. Learning to create such multidimensional formulations is an important step in avoiding the reductionist thinking that plagues much health-care delivery. No student should graduate thinking that assigning a diagnostic label is any more than a small part of understanding a patient.

Of all the elements—biological, psychological, and social—the least well integrated is the social. Yet the social situation of patients can have a major influence on their diagnosis and care. In Atkins's case, a sort of vicious circle appeared in relation to her social situation. The absence of her family members subtly reinforced the disengagement of health professionals: we still have a rather tacit expectation that there will be a functional and supportive family. For the health-care team, the absence of supports almost certainly reinforced the idea that Atkins was "difficult." It may have simultaneously aroused their fear that they were being "stuck" with a patient for whom there were few supports and to whom they had to provide even more. Instead of enhancing their curiosity, Atkins's lack of family support seems to have killed it entirely.

Atkins's nurses and doctors seemed to be as incurious about her new family as they were about her old one. Few of her caregivers seem to have had much curiosity or interest in any discussion of the significant joys and challenges that punctuated Atkins's life. Amazingly, while Atkins was so terribly sick, she managed to finish university, get a PhD, find a partner, and adopt children. These would be major accomplishments for any of us. Considering her condition, they are remarkable. Yet no one seems to have tried to harness these accomplishments for their therapeutic value. One can imagine that asking a few questions about such major developments as a new partner, academic accomplishments, adoption or birth of children would convey the curiosity that signals to patients that a healthcare professional is interested in them.

When I see curiosity failing in one of my students, I use an exercise that has proved very helpful over the years. This technique was taught to me by one of my teachers, Dr. Edred Flak. The exercise proceeds as follows: the student sits with a patient and has the patient recount their life story. The student takes notes, then goes away and writes up the patient's biography. The student then returns to see the patient and reads, or has the patient read, the narrative. The patient and student then discuss any omissions or problems of emphasis, and the student rewrites the story until the patient feels that it accurately captures his or her life. No student I have asked to do this has ever emerged from the experience without a rich and empathic understanding of the patient as well as a broader view of the many influences on the patient's illness. While a busy health-care professional will clearly not have time to write a patient's biography, the principle of every encounter should be the same: asking a few questions that will help understand the context and meaning of the patient's life. Who ever asked Atkins, "How does this illness affect your life?" In the health professions there can be no competence without curiosity.

Preserving Dignity and Establishing Trust

Perhaps the hardest of the three attributes to master is creating trust. Yet in Atkins's narrative we see that individuals who were able to create trust had much better interactions with her. There was, for example, the neurosurgeon that Atkins felt "treated me with what appeared to be genuine concern and respect." As result of this climate of trust, even when the surgeon declined to undertake the operation that Atkins wanted, she was able to accept his advice, noting that she "understood his qualms." Similarly, we read about an emergency room doctor whose frankness on several occasions "created trust."

Establishing trust stems, in part, from a concerted effort to maintain the dignity of people as they pass through the health-care system. In Atkins's narrative, the central role of dignity is always highlighted. She writes that "while many physicians remained dubious, there were a remarkable few who always treated me with dignity and who fought to save my life when others dismissed me as unworthy and incurable." Preserving dignity requires health professionals to know something about the patient, to engage in a curious and interested way, and to try to build trust. The antithesis of dignity occurs when the health-care environment fosters shame, guilt, or futility. Yet Atkins notes that many times, "even as I endured severe weakness and physical dependency and was classified as a palliative care patient, my suffering and needs were overshadowed by the specter that they were not, in fact, real, and that I was some sort of emotional con artist, intent on exploiting valuable medical resources and attention." Why is preserving patient dignity so hard? Is lack of preparation a factor? One of my own students, Dr. Glendon Tait, conducted a study of resident trainees' attitudes toward very ill and dying patients.[17] He found that, even in psychiatry, the next generation of doctors felt poorly prepared to address the existential, spiritual, and cultural aspects of patients' care, which are the very things that research tells us are most strongly aligned with patients' concepts of dignity.

To make matters worse, many things that seem bizarre and intrusive to patients have become "normalized" in health-care settings. Consider the simple act of putting on a "blue gown," that lovely piece of haute couture that barely reaches the knees and has a long slit up the back fastened with

17. Tait, G., Hodges, B. (2009) "End-Of-Life Care Education in Psychiatry Residents' Attitudes, Preparedness, and Conceptualizations of Dignity." *Acad Psych* 33, no. 6:451–56.

two ties, out of reach to anyone but a steady practitioner of yoga. How about the very common practice of bursting into a patient's room and just talking or examining the patient with no introduction? Can you imagine why a health professional thinks it is appropriate to barge into your room and, instead of telling you his or her name, uses a label to present him or herself? "Hi, I'm the on-call" or "I'm the resident" Somehow the strangeness of these practices is barely visible to most health professionals. Yet they dehumanize and objectify patients—as well as health professionals themselves—in a way that does nothing to build an atmosphere of trust.

Interestingly, every doctor I know who has had to change out of street clothes into a blue gown and sit in a hallway waiting for a test or appointment while the general public passes by experiences the shock and embarrassment of something they ask their patients do every day. This "turning of the tables," whereby a health professional becomes a patient, was dramatized in the 1991 Hollywood film *The Doctor* (starring William Hurt and Elizabeth Perkins and based on the book *A Taste of My Own Medicine* by Dr. Edward E. Rosenbaum). Used in many medical school curricula, this film helps make the gulf between what is done to patients and what it feels like to have these things done to oneself as a doctor more real for students. Some health-professional training programs go so far as asking students to give each other IVs, to require that students use wheelchairs or other assistive devices for a week, or to prick their own finger with a lance every four hours to measure their blood sugar. Certainly, these experiences help personalize illness and the indignities of treatment. Similarly, physicians and other health-care professionals who have themselves been through an illness are often more empathic, because they know that preserving patient dignity is essential for fostering trust. However, health professionals can learn to be attentive to the dignity of patients and to build a sense of trust if they develop the skill of objectifying the disease, not the patient.

Objectifying the Disease, Not the Patient

In order for treatment to advance, health professionals and the patient must be aligned in a mission *against something*. The language of "fighting" illnesses such as cancer illustrates this alignment. We speak about "the long battle with cancer," "the struggle with Parkinson's," or "the fight to survive." Hidden in this language is a key issue: for the fight or struggle to be effective the patient and his or her health-care professionals must be *in alliance*. They must be on the same side. Together they objectify the illness and target all their efforts toward defeating it.

However, what happened time and again to Atkins, and what is a risk for anyone diagnosed with a psychological component to their illness or who has a hard-to-diagnose illness, is that health professionals become allied *against the patient*. Because psychosomatic illnesses can never be completely attributed to an external cause (bacteria, lesion, tumor), fighting one creates a confused struggle that is, in part, a fight against the "self" of the patient. Atkins says, "Instead of my illness being the problem, I became the problem." Instead of fighting together *against* the illness, the patient was left feeling "fraudulent and delusional"—part of the problem, not the solution. This, as Atkins observes, "leads clinicians of all types to blame the patient for her symptoms and to view the symptoms as purely the purview of psychiatry." What sort of approach should health professionals take when confronted with hard-to-diagnose illness? It is difficult to form a therapeutic alliance if you don't know what you are fighting. First, we doctors and nurses must recognize our tendency to feel powerless in the face of uncertainty. However, a shared feeling of impotence will not help the patient. Instead, we must find something to ally with the patient against. That something, however, does not necessarily have to be a clear-cut, codified diagnosis from the *International Classification of Diseases* (ICD).[18]

I was fortunate early in my training to encounter a gifted colleague who specialized in the treatment of patients who fall into that space between medical and psychological illness. Dr. Susan Abbey's first lesson was that the binary of "either/or" should be avoided. She reinforced how important it was to acknowledge and respect both physical and psychological

18. *International Statistical Classification of Diseases and Related Health Problems*, 10th revision, 2nd ed. (ICD-10). (2004). Geneva: World Health Organization.

symptoms and to preserve patient dignity. She taught me to use the analogy of "carrying two heavy suitcases—one with the physical symptoms and one with the psychological ones," thereby objectifying both aspects of the illness and not the patient. Following this logic, both the doctor and the patient have two burdens to deal with simultaneously. Extending this analogy, the doctor might tell a patient something like, "On the one hand, you have the physical symptoms—breathing problems, weakness, spasticity—and, on the other, the psychological ones—frustration, depression, anxiety. These are like two heavy suitcases that you are carrying. We must look at both of them and see if we can find ways to lighten each of the loads."

Today many health professionals find that a helpful way of engaging patients in the struggle against their illness is to involve them in reading the medical literature. Patients and families often believe that once a diagnosis is found, treatments are well defined and agreed on. The rhetoric of "evidence-based medicine" encourages the notion that there is certainty. In fact, few diagnostic approaches are strongly evidence based, and most outcomes are highly variable depending on culture, gender, and age. The clinician must weigh the available evidence and creatively select from many options based on a combination of intuition, experience, and context. Much like an artist selecting from a range of paints to create a desired color, this mixing and choosing is the art of medicine. However, this process goes on largely in the mind of clinicians and is rarely discussed openly with patients or their families. Yet, as Atkins notes, with the dawn of the Internet age, patients have access to the same medical databases as their physicians. An effective way to engage patients in a shared fight against their illnesses is to help them understand and appraise the medical literature. It is true (I can hear the objections of my colleagues) that much of what is found on the Internet is questionable and that much formal medical literature is filled with jargon. Nevertheless, when patients, families, and members of the health-care team can "share their thinking," much of the energy of the struggle can be channeled into the challenge of fighting the illness rather than into a fight between the patient and the medical team. Atkins writes that she and Aruna "never really read through the materials in a sustained or methodical manner" but that when they did so, she became interested and reflective about the literature. Those with psychological training will identify this approach as "intellectualization," a process that can be helpful to both the health professional and the patient and that has the effect of distancing the emotional aspects of the disease in pursuit of a rational explanation and approach to defeating it.

Lessons for Health-Professional Education

While Atkins's narrative contains many lessons for those health professionals who are already in the workforce, many aspects of her experience shine light on particular problems in health-professional education. As I write this, both Canada and the United States are undergoing heated discussions about their health-care systems and are also rethinking their systems of medical and nursing education.[19] One hundred years have passed since Abraham Flexner's famous report restructured medical education in North America,[20] and while there have been improvements, there is growing awareness that the system has remained largely unchanged, leading to gaps in the competence of graduates. Atkins's experiences highlight some themes that need to be discussed in relation to the reform of both medical and nursing education.

Importance of Continuous Care of Patients
with Complex Problems

Anyone fortunate enough to have a family physician or family health team knows that ongoing care with one or more health professionals who get to know you and your family well enough to understand your

19. Association of Faculties of Medicine of Canada, *Future of Medical Education in Canada Project.* http://www.afmc.ca/projects-international-future-med-can-e.php (accessed Sept. 5, 2009). Josiah Macy Foundation, "Revisiting the Medical School Educational Mission at a Time of Expansion." http://www.josiahmacyfoundation.org/documents/ Macy_MedSchoolMission_proceedings_06–09.pdf (accessed Sept. 5, 2009).

20. Flexner, A. (1925). *Medical Education: A Comparative Study.* New York: Macmillan.

biological, psychological, and social issues and contexts is both comforting and essential to good care. Today, however, much care is delivered piecemeal by a series of individual consultants or professionals who see each patient only once or just a few times. Akins's experience illustrates the difference between a continuous presence and a parade of bit players. Atkins's encounter with a resident who had cared for her in the ICU speaks to the relevance of continuity of care to education. On meeting Atkins on the street he exclaims, "God, now I know we make a difference! I really thought you would die."

In my experience, medical students and residents rarely, if ever, get to see patients over time. The same is true of nursing and other professional students. While most illnesses have a course that waxes and wanes over months or years, most clinical rotations are measured in weeks. Exclusive exposure to small windows of time during which patients with chronic conditions change very little can lead to a pessimistic view about the likelihood of improvement. As a partial corrective to this problem, some medical schools are now creating longitudinal rotations in which students work with the same patients and teachers for a year or more. There is growing recognition that a string of experiences of two-to-four weeks does not help young doctors develop a realistic sense of the natural course of illness or an appreciation for the contextual, psychological, and social aspects of treatment and recovery. Similarly, some nursing schools are raising the same questions about nurses' episodic appearances in health-care institutions.

In particular, the central importance of strong relationships with families, social networks, and the identification of meaningful goals becomes visible only with more time with patients. Atkins tells us how her intimate relationships and her scholarly work gave her life a sense of meaning that helped her survive the darkest moments of her illness. It is said that the most important protective factor against suicide is hope, and we can see in this story that the most important element of hope for Atkins related to her relationships and her work. A clinician who cannot see this equation will be significantly less effective in helping patients. Medical, nursing, and other health-professional education must, then, continue to find models that expose students regularly and continuously to the longitudinal nature of illness, treatment, and recovery in the context of patients' lives and continue to move away from an overemphasis on very short "sampling"-type educational experiences.

Need for Certainty versus Tolerance of Ambiguity

Another problematic feature of modern medical education is a lack of training in tolerance of ambiguity. Something in the makeup of students and curricula seems to foster a need for certainty. Yet so much in health care is uncertain. While being able to make a rare diagnosis is a rewarding experience, somehow medical education fails to convey that most conditions remain undiagnosed and/or involve complex interactions of multiple problems. Atkins notes that when "confronted by a difficult and ambiguous case, most doctors and nurses routinely grasped for certainty rather than attempting to tolerate any ambivalence." I am among a group of health-professional educators who believe that this may be aggravated by the overuse of standardized cases in training and the reductionism that occurs when the assessment of competence is reduced to checklists. Both the Canadian and U.S. projects on the future of medical education have highlighted the need to give greater attention to understanding complexity and tolerating ambiguity. Says Atkins, "What I did not know was that medicine does not tolerate uncertainty very well. Medical personnel are trained to find a diagnosis."

The strong desire for certainty is a challenge in teaching. I recall one of my first-year students becoming frustrated when he found that three different books gave different values for the amount of drop in blood pressure that constitutes "orthostatic hypotension" (a condition that involves the dropping of blood pressure when one goes from lying down to standing). "This is what I can't stand about medicine; no one can ever give an exact answer," he said with frustration.

My student's comment made me wonder about the relative contributions of personality and training in learning to live with uncertainty. Certainly, intolerance of ambiguity does not afflict my friends in the social sciences or the arts. I realized in that moment that my response to this student would be important in his development as a doctor. I would have to talk to him about how he could learn to tolerate ambiguity and to overcome what Atkins calls "medicine's powerlessness in the face of uncertainty." The student appreciated that I came at the issue head on and noted that no one had taken the time to talk to him about this before. I connected his need to learn to tolerate ambiguity with the likelihood that if he didn't, he would get frustrated with patients and their problems. I asked him to think about why he felt such a strong need for certainty and what it might mean for him to work in situations where there was no possible correct answer. We also talked about how medical education trains students to "always have the right answers." He admitted that it would be hard for him to say "I don't know" during rounds. So here is the question: How can we teach our students to say "I don't know"?

Perhaps we can do this by emphasizing the definition of professional expertise conceived by the professors Carl Bareiter and Marlene Scardemalia.[21] These teachers define it as a willingness to engage, rather than to disengage, with complex problems and to embrace, rather than flee, ambiguity. It would seem that health-professional education must do more to embed this principle in training and practice.

Quality Is Just as Important as Quantity

There is no doubt in my mind that some readers will attribute the problems described in this book to lack of investment in health care; a shortage of doctors, nurses, and other health professionals; and the significant constraints on those who try to hold the system together. I cannot quibble with the reality of stretched resources or a shortage of personnel. What I would argue, however, is that most of the problems Atkins experienced were problems of quality of care, not quantity. Aside from problems with getting funding for a few assistive devices, she did not describe much difficultly in accessing an ambulance, getting to an emergency department, being admitted to a hospital, or getting appointments to see doctors and

21. Bareiter, C., and Scardemalia, M. (1993). *Surpassing Ourselves: An Inquiry into the Nature and Implications of Expertise.* Chicago: Open Court.

other health professionals. The problem for her was not access to care, but rather access to *the right kind* of care. Some might argue that her health professionals would have been more effective and compassionate if they just had more time. But would they? If we could double the number of doctors, expand the nursing staff, and add more rehabilitation therapists, would Atkins's experiences have been substantially different? It seems to me that the attitude toward her would have been the same, even with more personnel. How do we shift the focus from quantity to quality in health-professional education?

I was invited to observe a program meant to assist physicians with communication problems. While there, I watched an interaction between one of the course instructors and an obstetrician. The obstetrician felt frustrated that each time he was paged to leave his office to deliver a baby, he would return to a waiting room full of angry women who had been sitting there, sometimes for several hours, waiting for their appointments. He would frequently become embroiled in arguments with patients, who he thought didn't "appreciate what obstetrics is like." Further, he was not happy to be attending the communication course because he was certain that the main message was going to be "spend more time talking with patients." More time was one thing that he did not have. Surprisingly, the instructor told him something else: that he could teach him to take *less* time.

Surely, arguing with patients every time he had to pass through the waiting room was a waste of his time, the instructor remarked. The obstetrician heartily agreed. The instructor then went on to teach him that a well-placed apology and an acknowledgement that he understood the inconvenience, delivered to the people in the waiting room and reinforced in each appointment, would take only a few seconds but would save much time and frustration. Good communications is more often about quality, than quantity. Indeed, early in my training I had the great fortune to observe one of the most empathic physicians of my career—a surgeon who could convey a deeper sense of support, understanding, and empathy in five minutes than many physicians can convey in an hour.

It is in this sense that I suggest much of Atkins's problematic encounters could be improved without tripling the number of health professionals involved or morphing them all into psychotherapists ready to sit and talk for an hour. The key is to learn to replace frustration with curiosity (not "there is nothing wrong with you" but rather "I am puzzled by what is wrong with you"); to exchange hallway conversations conducted in the third person ("she's a nightmare") with direct communication ("I understand you have a very complex illness"); to add an inflection of honesty ("just like you, I find it frustrating that we cannot pin down a specific cause for these symptoms"); and to convey hope ("we will work together to do as much as possible to help you progress"). Done at every encounter, this need not take long: a few well-phrased words can diffuse the tension, ill will, and conflict that eat up not just minutes but hours of time. In an era when talk of cutting costs in the health-care system dominates all else, I wonder how much expense might have been avoided in Atkins's case if more efficient and effective communication had predominated.

Everyone's Judgment Is Compromised Sometimes

Let me illustrate this point and that made above with another personal experience. I was working in the emergency department one recent Friday afternoon. We had seen a lot of patients, and I was tired and keen to get home. As I was packing up my papers, my resident casually asked me if I had given any feedback to the medical student who had been working with us. Truthfully I had not, and was thinking that, given my fatigue, I might just skip it. But the resident persisted. Even though it was late, she reminded me that both she and I had noted that the medical student had a slight tendency to dismiss patients with serious psychotic symptoms. Earlier in the week, for example, he had recommended discharging a patient who was disturbed by hearing voices. Fortunately, medical students do not make decisions about admissions on their own, and I had chalked this up to a lack of experience. However, my resident thought that the student's dismissive attitude toward symptoms of mental illness should be addressed because it might signal a larger problem.

I called home to say I would be late and sat down with the student. At first he was defensive, noting that he was a top student and had received nothing but good feedback. We talked about his rotation and I wondered out loud if there might be something about some patients that made him feel he wanted to disengage from them quickly. He thought about it, but didn't say much. He seemed sullen as I described my worry that it might be dangerous if certain types of patients caused a reaction in him that he did not understand. He listened, nevertheless, and thanked me for my time.

About a month later I saw him by chance on a medical floor where he was doing his internal medicine rotation. He took me aside and told me that, though he could not tell me at the time we had talked, his sister had schizophrenia. As a child he had to endure watching her be restrained and hospitalized. After our conversation he realized how upsetting it had been for him to be in a psychiatric emergency department and confessed that he had just wanted to discharge everyone as fast as he could. I had earned the trust of this student on a day when I was nearly too tired to talk to him at all.

This experience illustrates several things that are relevant to the story Atkins tells. First, many health professionals have strong reactions to patients that arise, in part, from previous difficult or emotionally laden experiences with other patients, family, friends, or themselves. Second, we all reach a point when we simply cannot see—because of lack of time or fatigue—the need to intervene in a situation that we know deep down is problematic. Third, the effect of having a difficult discussion, be it between a health professional and a patient, two health professionals, or with a student may be delayed, and the results may not be immediately apparent. Nonetheless, these difficult discussions may often be transformative.

Even after years of training and practice in psychiatry, I am no master of my own emotions, nor do I always detect (as with this medical student) all of the nuances in the relationships around me. Therefore, it seems likely to me that most health professionals do not, and cannot, completely master the emotional domain on their own. Almost fifty years ago, Dr. Michael Balint described a technique that is unsurpassed today for mediating the effects of difficult clinical situations on physician judgment.[22]

22. The Balint Society. http://balint.co.uk/ (accessed September 5, 2009).

Widely held today, "Balint groups" engage a group of physicians in sharing and discussing their experiences with individuals they identify as challenging patients. In this shared space, the time, distance, and collective wisdom of colleagues allow for reflection and the identification of more productive approaches and behaviors. A tip I teach my students is that the minute they feel anger or frustration in relation to a patient or situation, it is a red flag that they should not ignore. They should go for a walk and when they get back make a date with a colleague to talk about the situation. Just as a night of "sober second thought" prevents many of us from sending ill-advised e-mail messages, a walk around the block and a chat with a colleague is the best way to avoid venting unhelpful emotions at a patient or their family.

Much attention is given today to the need for continuing education and the maintenance of competence. However, for many clinicians this consists of attending conference lectures on the latest in therapeutics. On the other hand, participation in a Balint-type group, where it is possible to reflect on and identify strategies for challenging situations, is more likely to improve patient care in the long run. I have participated in such a monthly study group since graduation from my residency program and see great value in being able to talk openly with colleagues in a supportive environment.

A Place for the Social Sciences in Health-Professional Education

In the 1960s, sociologists and anthropologists began to study health-professional education with great curiosity and produced books like *Boys in White*,[23] which opened the rather closed world of medical education to public scrutiny. While this work showed just how powerfully medical and other health-professional schools socialized their students into particular ways of thinking and behaving, the role of social scientists in health-professional education itself never blossomed. Today, medical educators

23. Becker, H., Geer, B., Hughes, E., Strauss, A. (1961). *Boys in White: Student Culture in Medical School.* Chicago: University of Chicago Press.

are once again recognizing that there is room for increased participation of social scientists in health-professional education.

There could be no better argument for the role of a social science perspective than this book. No one could read Atkins's narrative without seeing the central role of social context; professional socialization; health economics; and the constructed nature of illness, diagnosis, and treatment. All of these topics are of central importance and interest to the social sciences. It may well be that Atkins herself was able to write such a thoughtful and important narrative because she is now a professor of social science. The concepts she broaches, including the ways in which power is created and wielded by professions and institutions, the mechanisms by which health professions objectify patients, and the notion that illnesses themselves are fluid and co-constructed by the doctor and patient in an intersubjective space, are all powerful social science concepts that are almost unknown among health professionals.

Sociologists of medical education made an observation in the 1960s that is equally true today: solely changing health-professional education cannot change problematic behaviors that occur in health-care settings. The training period is too short and the workplace environment too powerful for lessons learned in medical or nursing school to endure. They must be systematically supported by changes in the workplace. Rude, intrusive, and objectifying behaviors will change when health professionals decide they are inappropriate in the workplace, not simply because they are taught in health-professional schools. But behaviors do change. Recently I saw a poster from the 1950s picturing a doctor promoting a brand of cigarettes. Today this seems strange and unprofessional. With social and peer pressure working in the right direction it is possible to change culture and to delegitimize problematic behaviors.

To conclude, Atkins's narrative is an informative and helpful corrective to some of the cracks and deficiencies in health-professional education, both at the individual level of learning and practice and at the systems level where the curricula and programs designed to train the next generations of health professionals are developed. The book is also a major contribution to showing why social scientists with expertise in the domains necessary to unravel the most troubling, complex, and ambiguous aspects of health, illness, and care should play a much greater role in health-professional education.

This book will raise the temperature of any health professional who reads it. However, having turned the last page, will any of us change our behavior the next time we go into the examination room, ward, or clinic? Indeed, I think this is possible—all the more so if reading the book can be accompanied by discussion and reflection with colleagues. For health-professional students and clinicians I have highlighted some ways to move from awareness to behavior change. Briefly these are:

- Learn to do a bio-psycho-social formulation, and incorporate it into patient charts and discussions.
- Try methods that objectify illness, not patients. The "two suitcase" analogy may be helpful where there are both biological and psychological components.
- Work toward healing the rift between physical and psychological aspects of illness.
- Learn some basic behavioral techniques and how to coach patients to use them.
- Focus on the quality of interactions rather than the time they take, emphasizing engagement, curiosity, and trust.
- Acknowledge the lack of certainty and even frustration, so long as a sense of hope is also conveyed.
- Become aware of feeling angry or frustrated, and talk to colleagues about patients and situations related to these feelings.
- Delegitimize behaviors that diminish the dignity of patients and families in the work environment.
- Keep focused on the question, how can I be helpful to this person?

To quote the popular alternative rock band Coldplay, health professionals need to ask reflectively and honestly, Am I part of the cure, or am I part of the disease? The professors Donald Schön and Ronald Epstein have argued that the ability to reflect on one's own thoughts, behaviors, and skills is central to medical competence.[24] As we see here, a clinician who has only a marginal awareness of his or her contribution to the construction of illness and its outcomes may inadvertently become more a part of the problem than part of its resolution. Each of us reading this narrative—whether health professional, patient, family member, or a general reader—might ask, how well would I cope in this situation? I am certain that the answer is as uncomfortable for the health-care professional as the doubt in the mind of a patient about whether she might be making some conscious or unconscious contribution to her own illness. We all do our best to keep such thoughts at bay. Nevertheless, health professionals and patients are together creating the "conditions of possibility" for every illness. Patients, families, and health professionals travel down the same road together. Atkins's moving work helps to remind us that it is a road better traveled when we are all facing in the same direction, with the same goal—the reduction of suffering in a context of curiosity, engagement, and trust.

24. Schön, D. A. (1987). *Educating the Reflective Practitioner: Toward a New Design for Teaching and Learning in the Professions.* San Francisco: Jossey-Bass. Epstein R. M. (1999). "Mindful Practice." *JAMA* 282, no. 9 (Sept. 1): 833–39.

Bibliography

Primary Sources

Atkins, Chloë. Journals. Unpublished, 1986–97.
Unspecified chart material. Unpublished, 1987–2000.
Wilmshurst, Rea. Journal. Unpublished, February 1995–March 1996.

Other Sources

Abrams, Kathryn. "Hearing the Call of Stories." *California Law Review* 79, no. 4 (1991): 971–1052.

Abse, D. Wilfred. *Hysteria and Related Disorders: An Approach to Psychological Medicine.* Bristol, UK: Wright, 1987.

Ainsworth-Vaughn, Nancy. *Claiming Power in Doctor-Patient Talk.* New York: Oxford University Press, 1998.

Appelbaum, Paul S., and Thomas Grisso. "Capacities of Hospitalized, Medically Ill Patients to Consent to Treatment." *Psychosomatics* 38, no. 2 (1997): 119–25.

Arboleda-Florez, J. "Reibl vs. Hughes: The Consent Issue." *Canadian Journal of Psychiatry* 32 (Feb. 1987): 66–70.

Aristotle. *The Politics.* Trans. Ernest Barker. Oxford: Oxford University Press, 1995.

Armstrong, Samuel Treat. "The Serum Treatment of Diphtheria." *Popular Science Monthly* (Feb. 1895): 512–22.

Ashe, Marie. "Zig-Zag Stitching and the Seamless Web: Thoughts on Reproduction and the Law." *Nova Law Review* 13 (1989): 355–83.

Barker, L. F. "The Antitoxin Treatment of Diphtheria." *Canadian Practitioner* 20 (1895): 99–101.

Barker-Benfield, Ben. "Sexual Surgery in Late Nineteenth Century America." *Journal of Health Sciences* 5, no. 2 (1975): 279–98.

Bate, Walter Jackson. *John Keats.* New York: Oxford University Press, 1963.

Bauby, Jean Claude. *The Diving Bell and the Butterfly.* Trans. Jeremy Leggatt. London: Fourth Estate Limited, 1997. Originally published as *Le scaphandre et le papillon* (Paris: Robert Laffont, 1997).

Beauvoir, Simone de. *The Second Sex.* New York: Alfred A. Knopf, 1953.

Berger, John. *Ways of Seeing.* Harmondsworth, UK: Penguin Books, 1972.

Biggs, Hermann M. "The New Treatment of Diphtheria." *McClure's* (Mar. 1895): 360–64.

Bloom, Hy, and Michael Bay, eds. *A Practical Guide to Mental Health, Capacity, and Consent Law of Ontario.* Scarborough, Ont.: Carswell, 1996.

Brody, Howard. *Stories of Sickness.* New Haven: Yale University Press, 1987.

Brown, E. Richard. *Rockefeller Medicine Men: Medicine and Capitalism in America.* Berkeley: University of California Press, 1979.

Broyard, Anatole. *Intoxicated by My Illness and Other Writings on Life and Death.* New York: Clarkson Potter, 1992.

Bruner, Jerome. *Actual Minds, Possible Worlds.* Cambridge: Harvard University Press, 1986.

——. "A Psychologist and the Law." *New York Law School Law Review* 37 (1992): 173–83.

Burke, Laura J., and Judy Murphy. *Charting by Exception: A Cost-Effective, Quality Approach.* Milwaukee: Aurora Health Care, 1988.

Burnum, John F. "The Misinformation Era: The Fall of the Medical Record." *Annals of Internal Medicine* 110 (1989): 482–84.

Califfe, Barbara. "Seven Things You Should Never Chart." *Nursing* (Mar. 1994): 43.

Caplan, Paula J. *They Say You're Crazy: How the World's Most Powerful Psychiatrists Decide Who's Normal.* Reading, MA: Addison-Wesley, 1995.

Cardinal, Marie. *The Words to Say It: An Autobiographical Novel.* Cambridge, MA: VanVactor and Goodheart, 1983.

Cassell, E. J. *The Healer's Art: A New Approach to the Doctor-Patient Relationship.* Philadelphia: Lippincott, 1976.

——. *Talking with Patients.* Cambridge: MIT Press, 1985.

Chatman, Seymour. *Story and Discourse: Narrative Structure in Fiction and Film.* Ithaca: Cornell University Press, 1978.

Diagnostic and Statistical Manual of Mental Disorders, 4th ed. (DSM-IV). Washington, DC: American Psychiatric Association, 1994.

Diagnostic and Statistical Manual of Mental Disorders, 3rd ed., text rev. (DSM-III-R). Washington, DC: American Psychiatric Association, 1987.

Diagnostic and Statistical Manual of Mental Disorders, 3rd ed. (DSM-III). Washington, DC: American Psychiatric Association, 1980.

Donne, John. "Devotions upon Emergent Occasions." In *Norton Anthology of English Literature.* Vol. 1, 4th ed. New York: W. W. Norton, 1979.

Donnelly, Strachan. "Human Selves, Chronic Illness, and the Ethics of Medicine." *Hastings Center Report* (Apr. 1988).

Donnelly, William J. "Righting the Medical Record: Transforming Chronicle into Story." *Journal of the American Medical Association* 260, no. 6 (Aug. 12, 1988): 823–25.

Ehrenreich, Barbara. "Sick Chic." In *Misdiagnosis: Woman as Disease*. Ed. Karen M. Hicks, 107–12. Allentown, PA: People's Medical Society, 1994.

Ehrenreich, Barbara, and Deirdre English. *For Her Own Good: 150 Years of the Experts' Advice to Women*. New York: Anchor/Doubleday, 1978.

Epstein, Julia. *Altered Conditions: Disease, Medicine, and Storytelling*. New York: Routledge, 1995.

Estrich, Susan. "Rape." *Yale Law Journal* 95, no. 6 (1986): 1087–188.

Evans, Martha Noel. "Hysteria and the Seduction Theory." In *Seduction and Theory: Readings of Gender, Representation and Rhetoric*. Ed. Diane Hunter, 73–85. Chicago: University of Chicago Press, 1989.

Feinburg, Leslie. *Trans Liberation: Beyond Pink or Blue*. Boston: Beacon Press, 1998.

Fink, Bruce. *A Clinical Introduction to Lacanian Psychoanalysis: Theory and Technique*. Cambridge: Harvard University Press, 1997.

Ford, Charles V. "Dimensions of Somatization and Hypochondriasis." *Neurologic Clinics* 13, no. 2 (1995): 241–53.

——. *The Somatizing Disorders: Illness as a Way of Life*. New York: Elsevier Biomedical, 1983.

Foster, W. D. *History of Medical Bacteriology and Immunology*. London: William Heinemann Medical Books, 1970.

Foucault, Michel. *The Birth of the Clinic*. New York: Pantheon Books, 1973.

——. *Discipline and Punish: The Birth of the Prison*. 2nd ed. Trans. Alan Sheridan. New York: Vintage, 1995.

——. *The Foucault Reader*. Ed. Paul Rabinow. New York: Pantheon Books, 1984.

——. *Mental Illness and Psychology*. Berkeley: University of California Press, 1987.

Frank, Arthur W. *At the Will of the Body: Reflections on Illness*. Boston: Houghton Mifflin, 1991.

——. *The Wounded Storyteller: Body, Illness, and Ethics*. Chicago: University of Chicago Press, 1995.

Freud, Sigmund. *Collected Papers*. Trans. Joan Riviere. 5 vols. New York: Basic Books, 1959.

Friedan, Betty. *The Feminine Mystique*. New York: Laurel, 1983.

Fugh-Berman, Adriane. "Man to Man at Georgetown: Tales out of Medical School." In *Misdiagnosis: Woman as Disease*. Ed. Karen M. Hicks, 47–54. Allentown, PA: People's Medical Society, 1994.

Gass, William. "The Art of Self: Autobiography in an Age of Narcissism." *Harper's* (May 1994): 43–52.

Gilligan, Carol. *In a Different Voice: Psychological Theory and Women's Development*. Cambridge: Harvard University Press, 1982.

Gilman, Charlotte Perkins. "The Yellow Wallpaper." In *"The Yellow Wall-Paper" and Selected Stories of Charlotte Perkins Gilman*. Ed. Denise D. Knight, 39–53. Newark: University of Delaware Press, 1994.

Gooch, Judith L., et al. "Behavioural Management of Conversion Disorder in Children." *Archives of Physical Medicine and Rehabilitation* 78 (1997): 264–68.

Good, Byron, and Mary-Jo DelVecchio Good. "In the Subjunctive Mode: Epilepsy Narratives in Turkey." *Social Sciences and Medicine* 38, no. 6 (1994): 835–42.

Good, Mary-Jo DelVecchio, et al. "Oncology and Narrative Time." *Social Sciences and Medicine* 38, no. 6 (1994): 855–62.

Greer, Germaine. *The Female Eunuch.* London: Flamingo Modern Classic, 1993.

Guthrie, Elspeth. "Emotional Disorder in Chronic Illness: Psychotherapeutic Interventions." *British Journal of Psychiatry* 168, no. 3 (Mar. 1996): 265–85.

Hacking, Ian. *Mad Travelers: Reflections on the Reality of Transient Mental Illness.* Charlottesville: University Press of Virginia, 1998.

——. *Rewriting the Soul: Multiple Personality and the Sciences of Memory.* Princeton: Princeton University Press, 1995.

Hilfiker, David. *Healing the Wounds: A Physician Looks at His Work.* New York: Pantheon Books, 1985.

——. *We Are Not All Saints: A Doctor's Journey with the Poor.* New York: Hill and Wang, 1994.

Horowitz, Mardi J. *Hysterical Personality Style and Histrionic Personality Disorder.* Northvale, NY: Jason Aronson, 1991.

Howse, Ena, and John Bailey. "Resistance to Documentation: A Nursing Issue." *International Journal of Nursing Studies* 29, no. 4 (1992): 371–80.

Hunter, Kathryn Montgomery. *Doctors' Stories: The Narrative Structure of Medical Knowledge.* Princeton: Princeton University Press, 1991.

Hyler, Steven E., and Robert L. Spitzer. "Hysteria Split Asunder." *American Journal of Psychiatry* 135, no. 12 (1978): 1500–504.

Hypatia: A Journal of Feminist Philosophy 7, no. 1 (Winter 1992).

Hysterie et obsession: Les structures cliniques de la neurose et la direction de la cure. Paris: Association de la fondation du champ freudienne, 1986.

Illich, Ivan. *Limits to Medicine: Medical Nemesis, the Expropriation of Health.* New York: Penguin, 1976.

Irigaray, Luce. *The Irigaray Reader.* Oxford: Basil Blackwell, 1991.

James, Alice. *The Diary of Alice James.* Ed. Leon Edel. New York: Dodd, Mead and Company, 1964.

Jennings, Bruce, et al. "Ethical Challenges of Chronic Illness." *Hastings Center Report* 18, no. 1 (Feb./Mar. 1988): S1–S16.

Johnson, Mark. *The Body in the Mind: The Bodily Basis for Meaning, Imagination, and Reason.* Chicago: University of Chicago Press, 1987.

Kardiner, A. *War Stress and Neurotic Illness.* 2nd ed. In collaboration with H. Spiegel. New York: Hoeber, 1947.

Katz, Jay. *The Silent World of Doctor and Patient.* New York: The Free Press, 1984.

Kay, Fiona M. "Balancing Acts: Career and Family among Lawyers." In *The Public/Private Divide: Feminism, Law, and Public Policy.* Ed. Susan B. Boyd. Toronto: University of Toronto Press, 1997.

Kermode, Frank. *The Sense of an Ending.* New York: Oxford University Press, 1967.

Kleinman, Arthur. *The Illness Narratives: Suffering, Healing, and the Human Condition.* New York: Basic Books, 1988.

Kleinman, Arthur, et al. "Culture, Illness, and Care: Clinical Lessons and Cross-Cultural Research." *Annals of Internal Medicine* 88 (1978): 251–58.

Kleinman, Charles S. "Turnabout." *Sciences* (Nov. 1987): 20.

Koch, Robert. *The Aetiology of Tuberculosis: A Translation from German of the Original Paper Announcing the Discovery of the Tuberculosis Baccilus.* New York: National Tuberculosis Association, 1932.

——. "Bacteriological Research." *British Medical Journal* 2 (1890): 380–83.

Konner, Melvin. *Becoming a Doctor: A Journey of Initiation in Medical School.* New York: Penguin, 1987.

——. "On Human Nature." *Sciences* (May 1988): 6.

Korpman, Ralph A. "The Computer-Stored Medical Record: For Whom?" *Journal of the American Medical Association* 259, no. 23 (June 17, 1988): 3454–56.

Kraggh, Helge. *The Historiography of Science.* London: Cambridge University Press, 1987.

Kristeva, Julia. *Les nouvelles maladies de l'âme.* Paris: Librarie Arthème Fayard, 1993.

Kroenke, Kurt, et al. "A Symptom Checklist to Screen for Somatoform Disorders in Primary Care Patients." *Psychosomatics* 39 (June 1998): 263–72.

Kuhn, Thomas S. *The Structure of Scientific Revolutions.* Chicago: University of Chicago Press, 1962.

Lakoff, George, and Mark Johnson. *Metaphors We Live By.* Chicago: University of Chicago Press, 1980.

Lerman, Hannah. *Pigeonholing Women's Misery: A History and Critical Analysis of the Psychodiagnosis of Women in the Twentieth Century.* New York: Basic Books, 1996.

Liebenau, Jonathan M. "Public Health and the Production and Use of Diphtheria Antitoxin in Philadelphia." *Bulletin of the History of Medicine* 61 (1987): 216–326.

Locke, John. *Second Treatise of Government.* Ed. C. B. Macpherson. Indianapolis: Hackett, 1980.

Luria, A. R. *The Man with a Shattered World: The History of a Brain Wound.* Trans. Lynn Soloroff. Cambridge: Harvard University Press, 1987.

——. *The Mind of a Mnemonist: A Little Book about Vast Memory.* Trans. Lynn Soloroff. Cambridge: Harvard University Press, 1987.

MacDonald, Michael. *Witchcraft and Hysteria in Elizabethan London: Edward Jorden and the Mary Glover Case.* New York: Tavistock/Routledge, 1991.

Magnus, Stephen, and Stephen Mick. "Medicals Schools, Affirmative Action, and the Neglected Role of Social Class." *American Journal of Public Health* 90, no. 8 (Aug. 2000): 1197–1201.

Mai, Francois. "Hysteria in Clinical Neurology." *Canadian Journal of Neurological Sciences* 22 (1995): 101–9.

Mann, Thomas. *The Magic Mountain.* New York: Random House, 1995.

Mansfield, Katherine. *Journal of Katherine Mansfield.* Ed. J. Middleton Murry. New York: Knopf, 1928.

Marques, Janice, et al. "Forensic Treatment in the United States: A Survey of Selected Forensic Hospitals–Forensic Treatment at Atascadero State Hospital." *International Journal of Law and Psychiatry* 16 (1993): 57–70.

Marx, Karl. "The Philosophic and Economic Manuscripts of 1844." In *The Marx-Engels Reader*. Ed. Robert C. Tucker. New York: W. W. Norton, 1978.

Masson, Mark S. *A Dark Science: Women, Sexuality, and Psychiatry in the Nineteenth Century.* New York: Farrar, Straus and Giroux, 1986.

Mastering Documentation. Springhouse, PA: Springhouse Corp., 1994.

Mathews, Holly, et al. "Coming to Terms with Advanced Breast Cancer: Black Women's Narratives from Eastern North Carolina." *Social Sciences and Medicine* 38, no. 6 (1994): 789–800.

Mayou, Richard, and Michael Sharpe. "Treating Medically Unexplained Physical Symptoms: Effective Interventions Are Available." *British Medical Journal* 315 (Sept. 6, 1997): 561–62.

Mazumdar, Pauline. "Immunity in 1890." *Journal of the History of Medicine* 27 (July 1972): 312–24.

——, ed. *Immunology 1930–1980: Essays on the History of Immunology.* Toronto: Wall and Thompson, 1989.

McCrum, Robert. *My Year Off: Rediscovering Life after a Stroke.* Toronto: Knopf Canada, 1998.

McDonald, Clement J. "Computer-Stored Medical Records: Their Future Role in Medical Practice." *Journal of the American Medical Association* 259, no. 23 (June 7, 1988): 3433–40.

Micale, Mark S. *Approaching Hysteria: Disease and Its Interpretations.* Princeton: Princeton University Press, 1995.

Miller, Nancy K. "Facts, Pacts, Acts." *Profession 92.* Ed. Phillis Franklin. New York: Modern Language Association of America [MLA], 1992, 10–14.

——. *Getting Personal: Feminist Occasions and Other Autobiographical Acts.* New York: Routledge, 1991.

Millett, Kate. *The Loony-Bin Trip.* New York: Simon Schuster, 1990.

Mravcak, Sally. "Primary Care for Lesbians and Bisexual Women." *American Family Physician* 4, no. 2 (July 15, 2006): 279–86.

Murray, James P. "New Concepts of Confidentiality in Family Practice." *Journal of Family Practice* 23, no. 3 (1986): 229–32.

Nedelsky, Jennifer. "Law, Boundaries, and the Bounded Self." *Representations* (Mar. 1990): 162–89.

——. "Meditations on Embodied Autonomy." *Graven Images* 2 (1995): 159–70.

Nuland, Sherwin B. *How We Die: Reflections on Life's Final Chapter.* New York: Random House, 1993.

Okin, Susan Moller. *Justice, Gender, and the Family.* New York: Basic Books, 1989.

Orr-Andawes, Alison. "The Case of Anna O.: A Neuropsychiatric Perspective." *Journal of the American Psychoanalytic Association* 35, no. 2 (1987): 387–419.

Palmer, Robert B., and Kenneth V. Iverson. "The Critical Patient Who Refuses Treatment: An Ethical Dilemma." *Journal of Emergency Medicine* 15, no. 5 (1997): 729–33.

Pasteur, Louis. "Lettre de M. Pasteur sur la rage." *Annales de l'Institut Pasteur* (1897): 1–18.

———. *Resultâts de l'application de la méthode pour prevenir la rage après morsure.* Paris: Gauthier-Villars, 1886.

Payer, Lynn. "Borderline Cases: How Medical Practice Reflects National Culture." *Sciences* 30, no. 4 (July 1990): 38–42.

Peele, Stanton. "'Ain't Misbehavin'." *Sciences* 29, no. 4 (July 1989): 14.

Pekkanen, John. *M.D.: Doctors Talk about Themselves.* New York: Delacorte, 1988.

Pinckney, Edward R., and Cathey Pinckney. "Unnecessary Measures: Physicians Are Relying Too Heavily on Medical Tests." *Sciences* 29, no. 1 (Jan. 1989): 20–27.

Pincus, Theodore, et al. "Social Conditions and Self-Management Are More Powerful Determinants of Health Than Access to Care." *Annals of Internal Medicine* 129 (1998): 406–11.

Plato. *Republic.* Trans. G. M. A. Grube. Indianapolis: Hackett, 1992.

Probyn, Elspeth. *Sexing the Self: Gendered Positions in Cultural Studies.* London: Routledge, 1993.

Rachels, James. *The End of life: Euthanasia and Morality.* New York: Oxford University Press, 1986.

Rawls, John. *A Theory of Justice.* Cambridge: Belknap Press of Harvard University Press, 1971.

Reich, Warren T., ed. *Encyclopedia of Bioethics.* 5 vols. New York: Macmillan, 1995.

Reif, Winifried, and Wolfgang Hiller. "Somatization: Future Perspectives on a Common Phenomenon." *Journal of Psychosomatic Medicine* 44, no. 5 (1998): 529–36.

Reiser, Stanley Joel. "The Era of the Patient: Using the Experience of Illness in Shaping the Missions of Health Care." *Journal of the American Medical Association* 269, no. 8 (Feb. 24, 1993): 1012–17.

Remen, Noami. *The Human Patient.* New York: Anchor/Doubleday, 1980.

Rice, Marnie E., and Grant T. Harris. "Ontario's Maximum Security Hospital at Penetanguishene: Past, Present and Future." *International Journal of Law and Psychiatry* 16 (1993): 195–215.

Roberts, Helen. *The Patient Patients: Women and Their Doctors.* London: Pandora Press, 1985.

Rosenberg, Charles E., and Morris Vogel, eds. *The Therapeutic Revolution: Essays in the Social History of American Medicine.* Philadelphia: University of Pennsylvania Press, 1979.

Ross, Robert R. *Time to Think: Cognition and Crime—Link and Remediation.* Ottawa: Department of Criminology, University of Ottawa, 1981.

Rothstein, William G. *American Physicians in the Nineteenth Century: From Sects to Science.* Baltimore: Johns Hopkins University Press, 1972.

Rozovsky, Lorne Elkin, and Fay Adrienne Rozovsky. *The Canadian Law of Patient Records.* Toronto: Butterworths, 1984.

Russell, Denise. *Women, Madness and Medicine.* Cambridge, UK: Polity, 1995.

Sacks, Oliver. *An Anthropologist on Mars.* Toronto: Vintage Canada, 1996.

———. *Awakenings.* New York: E. P. Dutton, 1983.

———. *A Leg to Stand On.* New York: Harper and Row, 1982.

———. *The Man Who Mistook His Wife for a Hat.* New York: Perennial Library, 1985.

Schelp, Earl E., ed. *The Clinical Encounter: The Moral Fabric of the Patient-Physician Relationship.* Boston: D. Reidel, 1983.

Sharpe, Gilbert. *The Law and Medicine in Canada.* Toronto: Butterworths, 1987.

Sheppele, Kim Lane. "Just the Facts, Ma'am: Sexualized Violence, Evidentiary Habits, and the Revision of Truth." *New York Law School Law Review* 37 (1992): 123–72.

Sherwin, Sue. *No Longer Patient: Feminist Ethics and Health Care.* Philadelphia: Temple University Press, 1992.

Shorter, Edward. *Bedside Manners: The Troubled History of Doctors and Patients.* New York: Simon and Shuster, 1985.

———. "The Borderline between Neurology and History: Conversion Reactions." *Neurologic Clinics* 13, no. 2 (1995): 229–39.

———. *From Paralysis to Fatigue: A History of Psychosomatic Illness in the Modern Era.* Toronto: Free Press, 1992.

Showalter, Elaine. *The Female Malady: Women, Madness, and English Culture, 1830–1980.* New York: Penguin, 1985.

———. *Hystories: Hysterical Epidemics and Modern Medicine.* New York: Columbia University Press, 1997.

Shrier, Ian, et al. "Knowledge of and Attitude toward Patient Confidentiality within Three Family Medicine Teaching Units." *Academic Medicine* 73, no. 6 (1998): 710–12.

Siegler, Miriam, and Humphrey Osmond. "The Sick 'Role' Revisited." *Hastings Center Report* 1, no. 3 (1974): 41–58.

Silverstein, Arthur M. "Cellular versus Humoral Immunity: Determinants and Consequences of an Epic 19th Century Battle." *Cellular Immunology* 48 (1979): 208–21.

Slater, E. T. O., and E. Glithero. "A Follow-up of Patients Diagnosed as Suffering from Hysteria." *Journal of Psychosomatic Research* 9, no. 1 (1965): 9–14.

Slavney, Phillip R. *Perspectives on "Hysteria."* Baltimore: Johns Hopkins University Press, 1990.

Smith, John M. *Women and Doctors: A Physician's Explosive Account of Women's Medical Treatment—and Mistreatment—in America Today.* New York: Dell, 1992.

Smith-Rosenberg, Carroll. *Disorderly Conduct: Visions of Gender in Victorian America.* New York: Alfred A. Knopf, 1985.

Speed, John. "Behavioural Management of Conversion Disorder: Retrospective Study." *Archives of Physical Rehabilitation* 77 (1996): 147–54.

Stark, Alex. "Innovation in the Design of the ICU: New Trends that Incorporate Patient and Family-Centered Design." *Minnesota Physician* (May 2004): 32–36.

Stone, Jon, et al. "Systematic Review of Misdiagnosis of Conversion Symptoms and 'Hysteria.'" *British Medical Journal* 331, no. 989 (October 29, 2005).

Strauss, Leo, and Joseph Cropsey. *History of Political Philosophy.* Chicago: University of Chicago Press, 1972.

Strouse, Jean. *Alice James: A Biography.* Boston: Houghton Mifflin, 1980.

Sulieman, Susan Rubin. *The Female Body in Western Culture: Contemporary Perspectives.* Cambridge: Harvard University Press, 1985.

Supeene, Shelagh Lynne. *As for the Sky Falling: A Critical Look at Psychiatry and Suffering.* Toronto: Second Story Press, 1990.

Taussig, Michael T. "Reification and the Consciousness of the Patient." *Social Science and Medicine Part B Medical Anthropology* 14, no. 1 (1980): 3–13.

Teasall, Robert, and Allan Shapiro. "Behavioural Interventions in the Rehabilitation of Acute v. Chronic Non-organic (Conversion/Factitious) Motor Disorders." *British Journal of Psychiatry* 185, no. 2 (2004): 140–46.

Thomas, Andrew M. "Patient Satisfaction: Measuring the Art of Science." *Journal of the American Medical Association* 280 (Dec. 23–30, 1998): 2127.

Todd, Alexandra Dundas. *Intimate Adversaries: Cultural Conflict between Doctors and Women Patients.* Philadelphia: University of Pennsylvania Press, 1989.

Tolstoy, Leo. *The Death of Ivan Ilyich.* London: Penguin, 1960.

Toops, Les. "Primary Care: Core Values: Patient Centered Primary Care." *British Medical Journal* 31 (June 20, 1998): 1882–83.

Tronto, Joan. "Beyond Gender Difference to a Theory of Care." In *An Ethic of Care: Feminist and Interdisciplinary Perspectives.* Ed. Mary Jeanne Larrabee, 240–57. New York: Routledge, 1993.

——. *Moral Boundaries: A Political Argument for an Ethic of Care.* New York: Routledge, 1993.

Veith, Ilza. *Hysteria: The History of a Disease.* Chicago: University of Chicago Press, 1965.

Wack, Renate C. "Forensic Treatment in the United States: A Survey of Selected Forensic Hospitals. Treatment Services at Kirby Psychiatric Center." *International Journal of Law and Psychiatry* 16 (1993): 83–104.

Waddie, Paul. "Column One: Broken Hearts: Crisis in the Cardiac Unit: Dr. Odim Came to Save Young Lives but within Months, 12 Children Had Died and Winnipeg Wondered Why." *Globe and Mail,* 27 Oct 1998.

Walzer, Michael. *Spheres of Justice: A Defense of Pluralism and Equality.* New York: Basic Books, 1983.

Warner, Judith. "Who's Protecting Bad Doctors?" *Ms.* 4, no. 4 (1994): 56–59.

Watson, Annita B., and Marlene G. Mayers. *Assessment and Documentation: Nursing Theories in Action.* Thorofare, NJ: Charles B. Slack, 1981.

Weintraub, Michael I. *Hysterical Conversion Reactions: A Clinical Guide to Diagnosis and Treatment.* New York: SP Medical and Scientific Books, 1983.

Wenegrat, Brant. *Illness and Power: Women's Mental Disorders and the Battle between the Sexes.* New York: New York University Press, 1995.

Wilbourn, Asa J. "The Electrodiagnostic Examination with Hysteria-Conversion Reaction and Malingering." *Neurologic Clinics* 13, no. 2 (1995): 385–404.

Williams, Patricia J. *The Alchemy of Race and Rights: Diary of a Law Professor.* Cambridge: Harvard University Press, 1991.

Woolf, Virgina. "On Being Ill." In *The Moment, and Other Essays,* 9–23. London: The Hogarth Press, 1948.

Yeazzell, Ruth Bernard, ed. *The Death and Letters of Alice James.* Berkeley: University of California Press, 1981.

Ziporyn, Terra. *Disease in the Popular American Press: The Case of Diphtheria, Typhoid Fever, and Syphilis, 1870–1920.* New York: Greenwood Press, 1988.

——. *Nameless Diseases.* New Brunswick, NJ: Rutgers University Press, 1992.

About the Authors

Chloë G. K. Atkins has a PhD in Political Theory and is currently an Associate Professor in the Law and Society Program at the University of Calgary. She has held Social Sciences and Humanities Research Council of Canada, Fulbright, Clarke, and Killam fellowships. Atkins publishes academic articles as well as fiction and nonfiction. Currently, she is writing a book on the difficulty of making ethical decisions in everyday life and drafting another on trust, human rights, and vulnerability. She is married and has four children. Atkins continues to be treated for "atypical myasthenia gravis"; both the disease and its treatment are not without ongoing complications; nonetheless, she draws pleasure, strength, and inspiration from her family and friends and from her passion for painting, writing, sports, and nature.

Brian David Hodges, MD, graduated from Queen's University Medical School in 1989, completed psychiatry residency at the University of Toronto in 1994, a Master's of Higher Education in 1995, and a PhD in 2007. Since 2003, he has been Director of the University of Toronto Wilson Centre, one of the largest centers for health professional education research in the world. From 2004 to 2008 he was Chair of Evaluation at the Royal College of Physicians and Surgeons, overseeing assessment in the sixty-two specialty programs in Canada. Internationally he has worked with medical schools and licensure organizations in New Zealand,

Switzerland, Poland, Japan, Jordan, Israel, France, China, Australia, and Ethiopia. In 2003 he spent a year at the University of Paris, earning a diploma in Health Economics and Social Sciences and established collaborations with the University of Paris and the École des Hautes Études en Santé Publique (EHESP) where he continues to serve as a member of the education board. He was named Full Professor and Richard and Elizabeth Currie Chair in Health Professions Education Research at University of Toronto in 2009.

Bonnie B. O'Connor holds a PhD in Folklore and Folklife from the University of Pennsylvania, where she focused her graduate studies on folk and popular systems of health care; health belief and behavior; and patients' expectations and experiences of health, illness, and care. During her twenty-one-year career in medical education, she has continued to research, publish, and teach in these and related areas, including complementary/alternative and integrative medicine, bioethics, and cultural/cross-cultural issues in health care and health communication. She is the author of *Healing Traditions: Alternative Medicine and the Health Professions.* O'Connor is currently Associate Professor of Pediatrics (Research) and Assistant Director of the Pediatric Residency program at the Warren Alpert Medical School of Brown University/Hasbro Children's Hospital in Providence, Rhode Island.

Index